COMPREHENSIVE REVIEW FOR
FMGEMS

The National Medical Series for Independent Study

COMPREHENSIVE REVIEW FOR
FMGEMS

John Bullock, M.S., Ph.D.

Associate Professor of Physiology
Department of Physiology
New Jersey Medical School
University of Medicine and
  Dentistry of New Jersey
Newark, New Jersey

Abdool S. Moosa, M.D., M.D.,
  B.Ch. (Rand), M.F.G.P. (SA)

Foreign Medical Graduate
Physician
Orlando, Florida

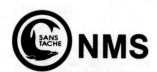

National Medical Series from Williams & Wilkins
Baltimore, Hong Kong, London, Sydney

Harwal Publishing Company, Malvern, Pennsylvania

Williams & Wilkins

The authors and publisher of this book have attempted to ensure that all recommended therapeutic modalities are in accordance with the accepted standards at the time of publication. The drugs specified in this book may not have specific approval of the Food and Drug Administration regarding the indications and dosages recommended by the authors. The best source of current prescribing information is the manufacturer's package insert, which should be consulted whenever possible.

Library of Congress Cataloging-in-Publication Data

Moosa, Abdool Sattar.
   FMGEMS/Abdool Sattar Moosa, John Bullock.
   p.   cm.—(The National medical series for independent study.
Exam series)
   ISBN 0-683-06216-6
   1. Medicine—Examinations, questions, etc.
   2. Physicians, Foreign—United States—Examinations, questions, etc.   I. Bullock, John,
1932-   . II. Title.   III. Title: Foreign medical
graduate examination in the medical sciences.   IV.
Series.   V. Series: A Williams & Wilkins medical
publication.
   [DNLM: 1. Foreign Medical Graduates—examination questions.   2. Medicine—examination questions.
W 18 M825f]
R834.5.M66 1988
610'.76—dc19
DNLM/DLC
for Library of Congress   88-11041
                                                      CIP

10 9 8 7 6 5 4

Dedications

To Fazila, Muhammad-Ameen, Yaaseen, and Hanief, for their support, encouragement, and perseverance.

To Barbara, who made it possible for me to complete two graduate degrees in physiology through her love and sacrifice. Included in this dedication are Laura, John, and Katherine, who also gave me reasons to pursue this endeavor.

To the many foreign medical graduates, who remain friends and colleagues.

To all scholars, who strive to increase their knowledge by learning and teaching, and to all teachers, who have given generously to their scholars their pearls of wisdom and knowledge.

Contents

Contents

Preface

In the writing of this examination review book, it was the authors' singular intent to provide the reader with the core of basic and clinical information that is representative of the new FMGEMS format. The approach that the authors used to determine the core of facts and concepts is based on experience—both academic and clinical—gleaned from 23 years of teaching in a school of medicine, 22 years of teaching review courses for foreign medical graduates, and 18 years of caring for patients in a general medical practice. We believe that these experiences have provided us with a realistic view of the examination requirements.

This test has been designed to provide the reader with an opportunity to determine areas of strength and weakness in clinical problem solving, using case histories from an active medical practice. The authors have attempted to achieve a balance in both the scope and the depth of the subject matter and in the variety of question formats. We believe that this book will allow the foreign medical graduate to prepare realistically for the current format of the FMGEMS examination, which appeared for the first time as a two-day examination in July 1984.

Although this text has been carefully referenced to the *National Medical Series for Independent Study*, the questions are not taken from that series. Thus, this publication provides both the doctor-student and the student-doctor with an opportunity for self-evaluation of his or her level of preparedness in a form that is truly novel.

John Bullock
Abdool S. Moosa

Acknowledgments

The writing, editing, and, most of all, the selection of medical subjects constituted a formidable task in order to provide a balanced work in terms of information and question format. To these ends, we herein recognize, remember, and laud Jane Edwards, who was the project editor for this book. It was Jane who served as the vis a tergo that led to the completion of the book.

We would also like to acknowledge the expert typing of the manuscript by Monica Veytie and the artwork of Marie Chartrand and Wieslawa Langenfeld.

We are grateful to Andy Ford and Jim Harris of Harwal/Wiley Medical for allowing us to tackle this project.

Introduction

Comprehensive Review for FMGEMS has been developed to help prospective examinees prepare for the Foreign Medical Graduate Examination in the Medical Sciences (FMGEMS). It should also be useful for individuals who are preparing for Part I, Part II, and the Federation Licensing Examination (FLEX) of the National Board of Medical Examiners (NBME) examinations, the Medical Sciences Knowledge Profile (MSKP), and the Medical Council of Canada Qualifying Examination (MCCQE).

A passing score on FMGEMS confers certification by the Educational Commission for Foreign Medical Graduates (ECFMG), allowing foreign medical graduates to: (1) obtain a visa to enter the United States, (2) receive graduate medical education (i.e., to enter a residency or fellowship program) in the United States, and (3) become eligible for licensure to practice medicine in the United States. FMGEMS replaces the ECFMG and the Visa Qualifying Examination.

FMGEMS, which is considered the equivalent of Part I and Part II of the NBME examinations, consists of 950 questions in the multiple-choice format. All of the questions are taken from the NBME test question pool. FMGEMS is given twice a year (January and July) on two successive days. The basic sciences are administered on day 1, and the ECFMG English test and the clinical sciences are administered on day 2. A passing score on the ECFMG English test is also required for ECFMG certification.

The NMS™ *FMGEMS* has been designed in accordance with the actual FMGEMS. It features 500 new questions, which are divided into two sections. **Section A** contains the basic science questions, covering the following subject areas: anatomy, behavioral science, biochemistry, biostatistics, histology and embryology, immunology, microbiology, pathology, pharmacology, and physiology. **Section B** contains the clinical science questions, covering the following subject areas: clinical pharmacology, medicine, obstetrics and gynecology, pediatrics, preventive medicine and public health, psychiatry, and surgery. **Section C** contains the correct answers and detailed discussions of the subjects raised by the questions. Each discussion, where possible, has been referenced to one or more of the NMS™ basic and clinical science review texts, including specific reference to the outline points under which the information necessary to answer the question can be found. Additional references are given in the Appendix.

Types of Questions

There are four different item (question) types used in this examination.

I. **Single best answer—single question**. This item type consists of a question or an incomplete statement followed by five answers or completions (options). The options are always lettered A, B, C, D, and E. The student is asked to select the *best* answer to the question. There may be other options that are partially correct, but there is only one answer.

   This item type usually examines the ability to complete a concept or provide a related fact. It is especially useful in identifying the most frequent or most relevant option from a list of occasionally or partially correct options.

II. **Multiple true-false questions**. This item type consists of an incomplete statement followed by four numbered answers or completions. The student is asked to determine whether each of the options is correct or incorrect; the answers are then given according to the following standard pattern, which allows for five different combinations. Mark

   A if **1, 2, and 3** are correct,
   B if **1 and 3** are correct,
   C if **2 and 4** are correct,
   D if only **4** is correct, or
   E if **all** are correct.

   This item type examines several related aspects of a particular topic.

III. **Matching questions**. There are two types of matching questions used in this examination.

   A. **Single best answer matching sets**. The first matching item type consists of *five* lettered options or a lettered diagram or illustration followed by a group of two or more numbered phrases or statements. For each numbered phrase or statement, the student is asked to select one option (answer) that is most closely related to it. Each option may be selected once, more than once, or not at all.

      This item type examines the ability to differentiate between concepts.

   B. **Comparison matching sets**. The second matching item type is a variant of the first. This item type consists of *four* lettered options followed by a group of two or more numbered phrases or statements. The student is asked to select a response for each numbered phrase or statement according to the following pattern. Mark

   A if the question is associated with **(A)** only,
   B if the question is associated with **(B)** only,
   C if the question is associated with **both (A) and (B)**, or
   D if the question is associated with **neither (A) nor (B)**.

   This item type examines the ability to compare and contrast two topics.

All of the items are arranged according to item type and are preceded by directions for that item type. The questions are randomly distributed within each of two sections (**A and B**) of 250 questions each.

It is suggested that approximately 1 minute be taken to answer each question; thus, there is a realistic 4-hour limit suggested for each section of NMS[TM] *FMGEMS*. This approximates the time constraints of the actual FMGEMS examination, which allows approximately 45 seconds for each question. If each section is treated as a separate test, only 4 hours need to be set aside at a time. If it takes less time to complete a section, the remaining time should be used to review that section just as in the actual test situation.

Section A

Anatomy
•
Behavioral Science
•
Biochemistry
•
Biostatistics
•
Histology and Embryology
•
Immunology
•
Microbiology
•
Pathology
•
Pharmacology
•
Physiology

Time—4 hours
Number of questions—250

QUESTIONS

Directions: Each question below contains five suggested answers. Choose the **one best** response to each question.

1. High levels of all of the following hormones are associated with diminished lower esophageal sphincter tone, decreased gastric motility, and increased secretion of bicarbonate and water by the pancreas EXCEPT

(A) gastrin
(B) secretin
(C) cholecystokinin
(D) gastric inhibitory peptide
(E) glucagon

2. Which of the following statements correctly refers to the epiploic foramen?

(A) It connects the middle ear with the inner ear
(B) The seventh cranial nerve traverses it
(C) The esophagus passes through it
(D) It is the opening between the greater and lesser peritoneal cavities
(E) The vagus nerve traverses it

3. Interferons are proteins that contribute to the natural immunity of the host. Their characteristics include all of the following EXCEPT

(A) they are inactivated by polymorphonuclear leukocytes
(B) they enhance T-cell (thymus-derived lymphocyte) activity
(C) they are produced by cells infected by viruses
(D) they induce the production of antiviral proteins that interfere with the translation of viral messenger RNA
(E) they potentiate the cytotoxic action of natural killer cells

4. A 38-year-old man complains of restlessness and irritability 3 weeks after the sudden death of his son who was killed in a motorcycle accident. He expresses anger toward his physician for not being available at the time of the accident, and he complains of numbness in both legs and paresthesia in the right palm. He is probably suffering from

(A) meningioma
(B) tabes dorsalis
(C) multiple sclerosis
(D) normal grief reaction
(E) cerebrovascular accident

5. Cholecystokinin is produced by the

(A) gallbladder
(B) liver
(C) pancreas
(D) stomach
(E) small intestine

Questions 6–8

6. A medical student examines a 45-year-old man presenting with a fixed facial expression and a "pill-rolling" tremor that is maximal at rest. Passive movement of the limbs gives the impression of "lead pipe" rigidity. The diagnosis that the student correctly makes is

(A) pseudobulbar palsy
(B) tuberous sclerosis
(C) sycosis barbae
(D) parkinsonism (paralysis agitans)
(E) catatonic schizophrenia

7. Which of the following occupations is most likely to predispose an individual to develop this condition?

(A) Plumber
(B) Carpenter
(C) Surgeon
(D) Boxer
(E) Golfer

8. Where is the lesion most likely to be?

(A) Occipital lobe
(B) Spinal cord
(C) Substantia nigra
(D) Optic chiasm
(E) Temporal lobe

(end of group question)

1

9. During the isovolumic contraction phase of the cardiac cycle, a number of events are observed including

(A) an increase in coronary blood flow
(B) the appearance of the second heart sound
(C) the appearance of the T wave of the electro-cardiogram
(D) a decline in aortic pressure
(E) the opening of the mitral valve

10. The patient in the photograph below presents with round lesions on the face and neck, which are increasing in size despite the application of cortisone cream given to her by a pharmacist. The diagnosis is most likely to be

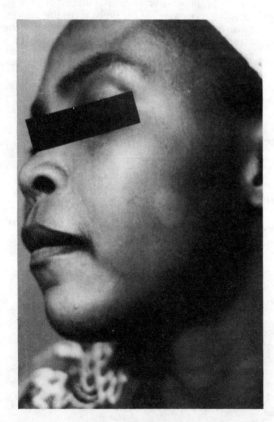

(A) pityriasis rosea
(B) nummular eczema
(C) candidiasis
(D) dermatophyte infection
(E) squamous cell carcinoma

11. The signs of a lower motor neuron lesion can include all of the following EXCEPT

(A) flaccid paralysis
(B) paresthesia
(C) paresis
(D) muscle atrophy
(E) hyporeflexia

12. Testicular function can be evaluated by the analysis of seminal fluid for

(A) prostaglandins, which are secreted from the prostate gland
(B) fructose, which is produced by the prostate gland
(C) acid phosphatase, which is released from the seminal vesicles
(D) citrate, which originates from the prostate
(E) ascorbate, which is produced by the prostate

13. The dorsalis pedis artery is the distal continuation of the

(A) peroneal artery
(B) medial plantar artery
(C) lateral artery
(D) anterior tibial artery
(E) lateral tarsal artery

14. The radius and the length of a tube are halved. According to Poiseuille's law, the resistance will

(A) increase by a factor of 8
(B) remain unchanged
(C) double
(D) fall to one-half of its original value
(E) fall to one-sixteenth of its original value

15. All of the following are classic examples of immune complex–mediated reactions EXCEPT

(A) serum sickness
(B) poststreptococcal glomerulonephritis
(C) erythroblastosis fetalis
(D) hypersensitivity pneumonitis
(E) Arthus reaction

16. Once formed, red blood cells normally have an average life span of

(A) 30 days
(B) 60 days
(C) 90 days
(D) 120 days
(E) 150 days

17. Which of the following changes occurs during isotonic contraction of a skeletal muscle?

(A) A bands shorten
(B) I bands shorten
(C) Z lines shorten
(D) actin filaments shorten
(E) myosin filaments shorten

18. Cerebrospinal fluid is produced in the ventricles by the

(A) choroid plexus
(B) dura mater
(C) myenteric plexus
(D) arachnoid villi
(E) none of the above

19. All of the following statements regarding syphilitic aortitis are true EXCEPT

(A) the essential lesion is an endarteritis obliterans of the vasa vasorum supplying the aorta
(B) it usually affects the ascending and transverse portions of the thoracic aorta
(C) it characteristically causes an angina that can be distinguished from other causes
(D) it occurs in the tertiary stage of the disease
(E) linear calcification limited to the roots of the aorta is a definitive diagnostic sign

20. Each of the following substances is a neuropeptide EXCEPT

(A) antidiuretic hormone
(B) thyrotropin-releasing hormone
(C) somatomedin
(D) oxytocin
(E) endorphin

21. All of the following statements regarding calcitriol are correct EXCEPT it

(A) is used therapeutically to treat hyperparathyroidism
(B) is a steroid with 27 carbon atoms
(C) is a metabolite of vitamin D_3
(D) is a secosteroid
(E) causes dissolution of bone

22. The lesion on the penis in the photograph below is caused by a

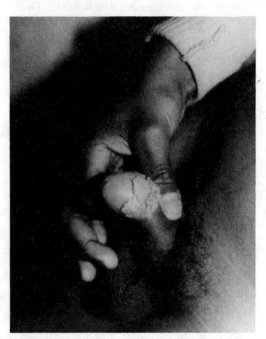

(A) spirochete
(B) papovavirus
(C) poxvirus
(D) retrovirus
(E) herpesvirus

23. Which of the following nerves or tracts contains upper motor neurons?

(A) Splanchnic nerve
(B) Supraopticohypophyseal tract
(C) Sciatic nerve
(D) Vagal efferents to the heart
(E) Vestibulospinal tract

24. Glycogenolysis in muscle does not contribute directly to blood glucose concentration because muscle lacks the enzyme

(A) phosphorylase
(B) phosphoglucomutase
(C) glucose-6-phosphatase
(D) glucokinase
(E) phosphoglucoisomerase

25. A patient who claims that he was a boxer by profession presents to you with "pill-rolling" tremor, rigidity, and hypokinesia. The lesion responsible for this condition is probably caused by

(A) heavy alcohol ingestion
(B) lesion in left temporal lobe
(C) petechial hemorrhages in the substantia nigra
(D) Brown-Séquard syndrome
(E) amphetamine abuse

26. Of all the phases of the menstrual cycle listed below, which four describe the same phase?

(A) Preovulatory, secretory, luteal, and progestational
(B) Preovulatory, proliferative, follicular, and estrogenic
(C) Preovulatory, proliferative, luteal, and progestational
(D) Preovulatory, proliferative, follicular, and progestational
(E) Postovulatory, secretory, luteal, and estrogenic

27. Typical features of trichinosis include all of the following EXCEPT

(A) convulsions
(B) eosinophilia
(C) muscle tenderness
(D) periorbital edema
(E) prodromal diarrhea, abdominal cramps, and malaise

28. The following information was obtained from a subject given a cardiopulmonary evaluation.

Heart rate = 75 beats per minute
Oxygen content in right atrium = 15 ml/dl
Oxygen content in pulmonary artery = 13 ml/dl
Oxygen content in femoral artery =
18 volumes %
Oxygen consumption = 300 ml/min
Hematocrit = 45%

The stroke volume (in milliliters) calculated from this data is

(A) 60
(B) 65
(C) 70
(D) 75
(E) 80

29. Propranolol administration may cause

(A) a rise in cardiac output
(B) tachycardia
(C) coronary vasodilation
(D) bronchodilation
(E) excitement and confusion

Questions 30–32

The effect of substrate concentration ([S]) on the velocity (V) of an enzyme-catalyzed reaction is summarized below.

[S] (mol/L)	V (nmol $\times$ L^{-1} $\times$ min^{-1})
3.33×10^{-6}	30
5.0×10^{-6}	40
1.0×10^{-5}	60
2.0×10^{-5}	80
4.0×10^{-5}	96
1.0×10^{-4}	109
2.0×10^{-3}	119
1.0×10^{-2}	120

30. The approximate Michaelis constant (K_m) for this system is

(A) 1.0×10^{-2}M
(B) 1.0×10^{-4}M
(C) 1.0×10^{-5}M
(D) 2.0×10^{-5}M
(E) 5.0×10^{-6}M

31. The estimated maximum velocity (V_{max}) for this enzyme-catalyzed reaction in mol $\times$ L^{-1} $\times$ min^{-1} is

(A) 40×10^{-9}
(B) 60×10^{-9}
(C) 80×10^{-9}
(D) 119×10^{-9}
(E) 120×10^{-9}

32. The K_m for an enzyme is 3.0×10^{-5} mol/L, and V_{max} is 5000 mol of substrate transformed per minute per mole of enzyme. What is the initial rate of the reaction at a substrate concentration of 3.0×10^{-5} mol/L in moles of substrate transformed per minute per mole of enzyme?

(A) 50
(B) 250
(C) 500
(D) 2500
(E) 5000

(end of group question)

33. All of the following clinical signs are associated with a lesion in the dorsal column EXCEPT

(A) astereognosis
(B) loss of temperature sense
(C) positive Romberg's sign
(D) loss of vibratory sense
(E) loss of two-point discrimination

34. A 40-year-old man presents with a "claw hand" deformity. This is probably due to a lesion of the

(A) medial nerve
(B) radial nerve
(C) brachial plexus
(D) ulnar nerve
(E) none of the above

35. Gamma efferent fibers are distributed to

(A) intrafusal fibers
(B) annulospiral endings
(C) vascular smooth muscle
(D) tendons of skeletal muscle
(E) cutaneous touch receptors

36. The formula below is that of

(A) epinephrine
(B) retinol
(C) vitamin D_3
(D) arachidonic acid
(E) prostaglandin E_2

37. Buerger's disease (thromboangiitis obliterans) has all of the following features EXCEPT

(A) it occurs exclusively in women
(B) it can cause gangrene
(C) it is associated with heavy smoking
(D) it involves arteries, veins, and nerves of the lower extremities
(E) the upper extremities are sometimes affected

38. The following pulmonary function data were obtained in a healthy subject.

Total lung capacity = 6.5 L
Functional residual capacity = 3.0 L
Vital capacity = 4.5 L

What is the expiratory reserve volume (in liters) of this subject?

(A) 0.5
(B) 1.0
(C) 1.5
(D) 2.0
(E) 2.5

39. Clinical vitamin B_{12} deficiency may be caused by all of the following EXCEPT

(A) regional ileitis
(B) gastrectomy
(C) fish tapeworm disease
(D) deficiency of "intrinsic factor"
(E) multiple polyposis (polyposis coli)

40. In the healthy kidney, which of the following substances has the lowest renal clearance?

(A) Urea
(B) Creatinine
(C) Inulin
(D) Glucose
(E) Potassium

41. All of the following statements regarding insulin are true EXCEPT

(A) it is synthesized by β islet cells of the pancreas
(B) it has no effect on protein metabolism
(C) it is a polypeptide consisting of two chains connected by two disulfide bridges
(D) it has no measurable effect on transport of glucose into brain cells
(E) it promotes glycogen synthesis by stimulating the actions of glucokinase and glycogen synthetase in the liver

42. The equation $pH = 6.1 + \log [HCO_3^-]/S \times P_{CO_2}$ is referred to as

(A) the Bohr effect
(B) the Henderson-Hasselbalch equation
(C) the Nernst equation
(D) Newton's law
(E) none of the above

43. Given the following data:

Mean capillary hydrostatic pressure = 32 mm Hg
Plasma oncotic pressure = 25 mm Hg
Tissue hydrostatic pressure = 4 mm Hg
Tissue colloid osmotic pressure = 6 mm Hg

the net force in mm Hg tending to move water from the capillary to the interstitial space is approximately

(A) 5
(B) 7
(C) 9
(D) 11
(E) 13

44. An individual has a ratio of total dead space to tidal volume of 0.25, a tidal volume of 0.8 L, and a respiratory rate of 10 breaths per minute. What is the alveolar ventilation in liters per minute?

(A) 1.2
(B) 2.0
(C) 3.3
(D) 4.8
(E) 6.0

45. In the heart, the term "increased afterload" can be used interchangeably with

(A) increased ventricular filling
(B) decreased ventricular end systolic volume
(C) increased aortic diastolic pressure
(D) increased ventricular contractility
(E) increased ventricular ejection volume

46. Drugs that are contraindicated during pregnancy because of their likely teratogenic effects include all of the following EXCEPT

(A) alcohol
(B) tetracycline
(C) vitamin A
(D) lithium
(E) penicillin

47. A patient with anemia would be expected to have

(A) an increased plasma concentration of bicarbonate
(B) an increased oxygen capacity of the blood
(C) an increased oxygen content of the blood
(D) a decreased arterial oxygen tension
(E) a decreased concentration of carbaminohemoglobin

48. A subject's tritiated water space was found to be 50 L of which the inulin space was 20 L with an osmolality of 300 mOsm/L. What will be the steady state osmolality (mOsm/L) of the intracellular fluid compartment if this subject drinks sufficient pure water to expand the extracellular fluid (ECF) volume by 5 L?

(A) 164
(B) 273
(C) 300
(D) 324
(E) The osmolality of the ECF cannot be determined

49. Pulmonary airway resistance is

(A) located mainly in the airways less than 1 mm in diameter
(B) higher on forced expiration than forced inspiration
(C) increased by alveolar hypoxia
(D) increased following atropine administration
(E) increased at high lung volumes

50. The renal mechanism for hydrogen ion excretion with the greatest capacity for increased activity during acidotic states is

(A) titratable acid excretion
(B) sulfate excretion
(C) ammonia trapping
(D) monobasic sodium phosphate excretion
(E) dibasic sodium phosphate excretion

Directions: Each question below contains four suggested answers of which **one or more** is correct. Choose the answer

A if **1, 2, and 3** are correct
B if **1 and 3** are correct
C if **2 and 4** are correct
D if **4** is correct
E if **1, 2, 3, and 4** are correct

51. A volunteer who was placed on a long-term diet containing a daily sodium intake of 30 mEq was treated by a drug that completely blocks the angiotensin-converting enzyme. The physiologic responses that are likely to occur during the subsequent hour include

(1) decreased mean arterial blood pressure
(2) increased sodium reabsorption by the distal convoluted tubule
(3) increased renin secretion
(4) increased plasma concentration of angiotensin II

52. Characteristics of chronic active hepatitis include which of the following?

(1) It is associated with hepatitis B
(2) It is more prevalent in postmenopausal women
(3) Most cases are idiopathic
(4) It involves inflammation of the liver that as a rule resolves in 3 months

53. Which of the following drugs may cause a lupus erythematosus–like syndrome?

(1) Hydralazine
(2) Phenytoin
(3) Procainamide
(4) Prednisone

54. The P_{50} for blood with a pH of 7.4 and a P_{CO_2} of 40 mm Hg is about 27 mm Hg. Under which of the following conditions would the P_{50} be increased above this normal value?

(1) Increased 2,3-diphosphoglycerate concentration
(2) Metabolic acidosis
(3) Temperature increase
(4) Hypercapnea

55. A patient who is withdrawing from opioids is likely to present with

(1) rhinorrhea and lacrimation
(2) yawning
(3) piloerection
(4) severe hypotension

56. Heparin, a mixture of highly electronegative sulfated mucopolysaccharides, has which of the following properties?

(1) It is a vitamin K antagonist
(2) It is an antiplatelet drug
(3) It is a fibrinolytic agent
(4) It has no effect on the synthesis of blood coagulation factors

57. The formation of a hypertonic urine is determined by a number of renal processes including

(1) the active reabsorption of water by the collecting ducts
(2) the formation of a hypertonic medullary interstitium by the reabsorption of sodium chloride and urea
(3) the passive reabsorption of water from the thin and thick segments of the ascending limb of the loop of Henle
(4) the increase in the water and urea permeability of the medullary collecting ducts by antidiuretic hormone

58. Correct statements about Babinski's reflex include which of the following?

(1) It is normally present up to 18 months of age
(2) It involves the flexion of the extremities in response to sudden stimulation
(3) It suggests an upper motor neuron lesion if present in an adult
(4) It excludes an upper motor neuron lesion if absent in an adult

59. The daily administration of a single small dose of 300 mg of aspirin can be associated with the

(1) irreversible inhibition of platelet cyclooxygenase
(2) prolongation of bleeding time
(3) inhibition of prostaglandin synthesis
(4) blockade of thromboxane A_2 synthesis

60. The accommodative reflex, which is activated when objects are moved closer to the eyes, includes

(1) convergence of the eyes
(2) thickening of the lens
(3) contraction of the pupillary sphincter
(4) contraction of the ciliary muscles of the eye

61. Complete median nerve paralysis in the axilla produces

(1) weakness of abduction of the thumb
(2) inability to pronate the forearm
(3) loss of light touch sensation over the palmar aspect of the index finger
(4) wasting of the hypothenar eminence

62. Adrenomedullary hormone secretion is described by which of the following statements?

(1) It requires an intact nerve supply
(2) It is stimulated by parasympathetic fibers
(3) It requires the secretion of acetylcholine
(4) It is mainly in the form of norepinephrine

63. During fasting, the substances that are important for gluconeogenesis include

(1) pyruvate
(2) glycerol
(3) lactate
(4) amino acids

64. Digitalis, a cardiac glycoside, is used in the treatment of congestive heart failure and tachycardia of supraventricular (atrial) origin. Cardiac glycosides have the unique ability to act directly on the myocardium to increase contractility. The untoward cardiac effects of digitalis intoxication can

(1) result in the initiation and maintenance of tachyarrhythmias
(2) be, in part, due to myocardial ischemia
(3) be associated with intracellular accumulation of sodium ion (Na^+) and loss of potassium ion (K^+) due to inhibition of Na^+, K^+–adenosine triphosphatase
(4) be potentiated by propranolol

65. The sound of 10,000 Hz falling on the ear leads to a number of auditory responses including

(1) oscillations in the basilar membrane beginning at the round window
(2) oscillations of the fluids (i.e., perilymph) in the cochlea
(3) oscillation of the basilar membrane throughout its entire length
(4) maximum oscillation of the basilar membrane near the base of the cochlea

66. Gallbladder contraction is stimulated by

(1) parasympathetic stimulation
(2) gastrin
(3) glucagon
(4) cholecystokinin

67. A plasma bicarbonate level of 32 mEq/L is consistent with

(1) persistent vomiting due to pyloric stenosis
(2) chronic renal failure
(3) hypokalemia
(4) diabetic ketoacidosis

68. "Privileged tissues," which are used for grafting because they are never rejected irrespective of where they are transplanted, include which of the following?

(1) Bone
(2) Skin
(3) Cartilage
(4) Bone marrow

69. Giardiasis, caused by the parasite *Giardia lamblia*, is more common in

(1) children as compared to adults
(2) homosexual men
(3) patients with hypogammaglobulinemia and IgA deficiency
(4) patients with duodenal ulceration

70. Responses mediated by the activation of α-adrenergic receptors in humans include

(1) contraction of ciliary muscle
(2) contraction of the pupillary sphincter
(3) ocular convergence
(4) mydriasis

71. The carcinoid syndrome has which of the following features?

(1) It manifests with a symptom complex consisting of episodic flushing of skin, abdominal cramps, diarrhea, and asthma
(2) It is probably caused by a serotonin-secreting argentaffin tumor that has metastasized to the liver
(3) The primary tumor is most commonly located in the terminal ileum
(4) If it occurs in the appendix, it is usually benign and nonfunctioning

72. Zinc deficiency is usually associated with

(1) hypogeusia
(2) hypogonadism
(3) poor wound healing
(4) hyperphagia

73. Undesirable effects of mafenide, which is used in the treatment of extensive burns, include

(1) pain
(2) carbonic anhydrase inhibition
(3) metabolic acidosis
(4) delayed epithelialization

74. The following data were obtained during a renal function test of a healthy man.

Creatinine clearance = 150 L/day
Plasma creatinine concentration = 1.0 mg/dl
Urinary excretion of creatinine = 1700 mg/day

From these data, it can be concluded that

(1) glomerular filtration rate is 150 L/day
(2) creatinine is filtered and secreted
(3) the filtered load of creatinine is 1500 mg/day
(4) creatinine clearance is not a good index of renal function

SUMMARY OF DIRECTIONS

A	B	C	D	E
1, 2, 3 only	1, 3 only	2, 4 only	4 only	All are correct

75. Signs of an upper motor neuron lesion include

(1) contralateral spasticity
(2) contralateral loss of abdominal and cremasteric reflexes
(3) normal reactions to galvanic and faradic currents
(4) fasciculations

76. Colchicine has which of the following properties?

(1) It inhibits chemotaxis of leukocytes
(2) A major untoward effect is diarrhea
(3) Bone marrow suppression can occur with high doses
(4) It should be administered intramuscularly

77. Acute acetaminophen (paracetamol) poisoning may result in

(1) hepatic necrosis
(2) hyperventilation
(3) prolongation of prothrombin time
(4) gastric bleeding

78. Opsonization enhances phagocytosis by the presence of opsonins in serum, which include

(1) C3b
(2) fibronectin
(3) tuftsin
(4) beta lysin

79. Histopathologic changes that result from chronic inorganic lead poisoning include

(1) deposition of lead in osseous tissue
(2) basophilic stippling of erythrocytes
(3) segmental demyelination and axonal degeneration
(4) pulmonary interstitial fibrosis

80. During exercise, the trained athlete as compared to a normal untrained adult usually has

(1) a slower heart rate
(2) augmented cardiovascular efficiency due to enhanced oxygen delivery to active tissues
(3) a greater blood flow to skeletal muscle per unit mass of muscle tissue for the same amount of physical work done
(4) elevated resting blood pressure due to quadrichamber enlargement and myocardial hypertrophy

81. Which of the following biochemical or physiologic responses can be attributed to epinephrine?

(1) It causes glycogenolysis in liver and muscle
(2) It stimulates secretion of glucagon
(3) It increases coronary blood flow
(4) It has a predominant β-adrenergic effect on the pancreatic β cells

82. Characteristically, patients with neurofibromatosis may present with

(1) café au lait spots
(2) fibrous molluscum
(3) Lisch nodules
(4) polyposis coli

83. A cotransport mechanism is used to permeate the plasma membrane in

(1) glucose transport into the intestinal mucosa
(2) sodium influx into the cardiac cells
(3) glucose transport from the renal tubular lumen
(4) glucose transport into the erythrocyte

84. Correct statements concerning Moro's reflex include which of the following?

(1) If it is absent in neonates, it suggests central nervous system pathology
(2) It involves hyperextension and spreading of the toes in response to stroking the foot
(3) It may be associated with mental retardation and brain damage if present in an infant older than 9 months
(4) It is normally present in infants up to 3 months of age

85. Ventricular tachycardia may be treated with

(1) electrical cardioversion
(2) lidocaine
(3) procainamide
(4) phenytoin

86. Primidone, a drug used to treat convulsive disorders, has a number of adverse side effects including

(1) systemic lupus erythematosus
(2) hirsutism
(3) central nervous system depression
(4) hypertrophy of the gums

87. Sarcoma of the breast has which of the following features?

(1) It is a fairly common malignant neoplasm
(2) It spreads rapidly to the lymphatics
(3) It has poor results even if treated by radical excision
(4) It usually presents as a soft mass with prominent overlying vessels

88. The lymph node is characterized by the

(1) afferent lymphatics
(2) efferent lymphatics that leave at the hilus
(3) medullary cords composed of dense lymphoid tissue, lymphocytes, and plasma cells
(4) indented hilus through which the main blood supply courses

89. Meissner's corpuscles are found in abundance in the

(1) tips of fingers and toes
(2) palms and soles
(3) glans penis and prepuce
(4) duodenum and jejunum

90. Prostaglandins belong to a family of endogenous substances called eicosanoids. Correct statements about these substances include which of the following?

(1) They are synthesized in nearly all tissues
(2) They are derivatives of arachidonic acid
(3) They are synthesized in higher amounts following even slight tissue trauma
(4) They are stored in the liver

91. Somatostatin is a hormone that is

(1) secreted by the δ cells of the endocrine pancreas
(2) a tetradecapeptide
(3) secreted by cells of the gastrointestinal tract
(4) a potent stimulator of insulin secretion

92. Characteristics of T lymphocytes include which of the following?

(1) They are produced by the thymus-dependent system
(2) They produce antibodies
(3) They have a long life span (of months or years)
(4) They are phagocytic

93. Digitalis toxicity should be suspected in a patient taking digitalis who presents with

(1) nausea, anorexia, and vomiting
(2) xanthopsia, blurred vision, or visions of flashing lights
(3) confusion and disorientation
(4) Sydenham's chorea

94. Aspects of psychological development between 18 months and 3 years include

(1) play
(2) autonomy
(3) self-awareness
(4) gender identity

95. The following values were obtained from a sample of arterial blood from a patient undergoing pulmonary evaluation.

pH = 7.61
P_{CO_2} = 20 mm Hg
P_{O_2} = 40 mm Hg
Bicarbonate concentration ($[HCO_3^-]$) = 19 mEq/L

These findings indicate

(1) a $[HCO_3^-]$ to ($S \times P_{CO_2}$) ratio below normal
(2) a partial compensation of this acid–base imbalance
(3) an hypemic hypoxia
(4) a respiratory alkalosis

96. Correct statements regarding cromolyn in the treatment of asthma include which of the following?

(1) It prevents the release of mediators of bronchospasm from mast cells
(2) It is a potent H_1-receptor antagonist
(3) It is ineffective in the management of an acute attack of asthma
(4) It relaxes bronchial smooth muscle

97. Typical features of severe trichuriasis infestation include

(1) splinter hemorrhages
(2) thousands of barrel-shaped eggs in a stool
(3) muscle tenderness and periorbital edema
(4) dyspepsia and rectal prolapse

98. The amenorrhea that occurs during menopause is caused by the inability of the

(1) anterior pituitary to synthesize or secrete gonadotropins
(2) myometrium to respond to estradiol
(3) endometrium to respond to progesterone
(4) ovaries to respond to gonadotropins

99. Adverse drug interactions may occur if monoamine oxidase inhibitors are simultaneously administered with which of the following drugs?

(1) Isoproterenol
(2) Barbiturates
(3) Amitriptyline
(4) Propranolol

100. Correct statements regarding iron metabolism include which of the following?

(1) Active areas of iron absorption are the duodenum and upper jejunum
(2) Intoxication with oral iron produces gastrointestinal bleeding, drowsiness, acidosis, and delayed liver failure
(3) Absorption of inorganic iron is increased by vitamin C
(4) In the absence of menstruation, iron loss from the body is about 10 mg per day

101. Hypernephroma can present clinically as

(1) painless hematuria
(2) vena caval occlusion
(3) fever
(4) hypocalcemia

102. Correct statements concerning cardiac output include which of the following?

(1) At rest it is approximately 5 L/min in a normal adult
(2) It can increase to about 15–20 L/min with maximal exercise
(3) It is the product of stroke volume and heart rate
(4) It can increase up to 30 L/min in trained athletes during exercise

103. Peripheral VII nerve palsy (Bell's palsy) may result in

(1) ageusia in the anterior two-thirds of the tongue
(2) hyperacusis
(3) impaired lacrimation
(4) contralateral facial muscle weakness

104. Quinidine, an isomer of quinine and a major alkaloid of the chinchona tree, shares all the pharmacologic properties of quinine, in that it is antimalarial, antipyretic, ototoxic, and a skeletal muscle relaxant. Cardiovascular effects of this antiarrhythmic agent include

(1) hypotension
(2) atrioventricular block
(3) prolongation of the PR, QRS, and QT intervals
(4) myocardial depression

105. Melanin pigment is normally found in the

(1) uveal tract of the eye
(2) leptomeninges
(3) basal layer of the epidermis
(4) zona pellucida

106. Which of the following statements can describe the normal distribution of alveolar ventilation and blood flow in the lungs of a subject in the sitting or standing position?

(1) The blood flow per unit lung volume is lowest at the base
(2) The ventilation–perfusion ratio is highest at the base
(3) Ventilation per unit lung volume is highest at the apex
(4) The alveolar P_{O_2} is highest at the apex

107. Which of the following drugs may induce parkinsonism?

(1) Trifluoperazine
(2) Haloperidol
(3) Metoclopramide
(4) Amantadine

108. Characteristics of the conjugation of bilirubin include which of the following?

(1) It is deficient in the premature infant
(2) It is aided by sulfonamides
(3) It is catalyzed by glucuronyl transferase
(4) It takes place in the Kupffer's cells of the liver

109. The following data were obtained from a volunteer subject to the renal research laboratory for a baseline study of renal function.

	Plasma (arterial)	Plasma (venous)	Urine
Inulin	1.25 mg/ml	1.00 mg/ml	150 mg/ml
Glucose	...	80 mg/dl	...

Urine flow ($\dot{V}$) = 1.1 ml/min
Hematocrit = 45%

With reference to this data, correct measurements of renal function include

(1) glomerular filtration = 132 ml/min
(2) filtered load of glucose = 106 mg/min
(3) renal blood flow = 1200 ml/min
(4) filtration fraction = 0.11

110. Correct statements regarding fibrinolytic therapy with urokinase or streptokinase include which of the following?

(1) It involves the activation of the proenzyme plasminogen to the proteolytic enzyme plasmin, which degrades fibrin
(2) It should not be administered in the presence of streptococcal infections
(3) It can produce lysis of emboli and thrombi in both veins and arteries
(4) It should be monitored by measurement of the thrombin clotting time

111. Renin secretion occurs primarily from the

(1) afferent arterioles
(2) renal cortex
(3) juxtaglomerular cells
(4) macula densa cells

112. Methyldopa may cause which of the following untoward side effects?

(1) Sodium retention
(2) Galactorrhea
(3) Impotence
(4) Liver damage

SUMMARY OF DIRECTIONS

A	B	C	D	E
1, 2, 3 only	1, 3 only	2, 4 only	4 only	All are correct

113. Factors favoring glucose mobilization include

(1) low plasma glucose concentration
(2) glucagon
(3) an adequate supply of substrate for gluconeogenesis
(4) insulin

114. Examples of electrotonic potentials include

(1) phase 4 depolarization of the sinoatrial node
(2) a miniature end-plate potential
(3) an inhibitory postsynaptic potential
(4) the wave of depolarization in the myocardium

115. According to the Henderson-Hasselbalch equation, it can be concluded that

(1) the greater the concentration of dissolved carbon dioxide ($[CO_2]$) in plasma, the lower the plasma pH
(2) the $[S \times CO_2]$ content can be determined by summing the concentration of bicarbonate ($[HCO_3^-]$) and $[CO_2]$
(3) the greater the $[HCO_3^-]$ in plasma, the higher the plasma pH
(4) the pK is not an important factor in the calculation of pH of body fluids

116. Carcinoma of the breast is more common in the

(1) right breast
(2) left breast
(3) lower outer quadrant
(4) upper outer quadrant

117. Goitrogenic drugs include which of the following?

(1) Phenylbutazone
(2) Para-aminosalicylic acid
(3) Lithium
(4) Propranolol

118. Thiamine deficiency (beriberi) can cause

(1) diarrhea
(2) heart failure
(3) dermatitis
(4) polyneuropathy

119. Warfarin has which of the following properties?

(1) It is the most widely used oral anticoagulant
(2) It is not fetotoxic and thus is safe for pregnant women
(3) It effectively inhibits the hepatic synthesis of vitamin K–dependent coagulation factors
(4) it potentiates the action of vitamin K on the fibrinolytic system

120. Hormones that stimulate glycogenolysis include

(1) cortisol
(2) glucagon
(3) insulin
(4) epinephrine

121. Correct statements regarding the neurotransmitters of the autonomic nervous system include which of the following?

(1) All preganglionic neurons are cholinergic
(2) Postganglionic parasympathetic neurons are cholinergic
(3) Sweat glands are innervated by postganglionic sympathetic cholinergic neurons
(4) The adrenal medulla is innervated by adrenergic fibers of the sympathetic nervous system

Directions: The groups of questions below consist of lettered choices followed by several numbered items. For each numbered item, select the one lettered choice with which it is most closely associated. Each lettered choice may be used once, more than once, or not at all. Choose the answer

A if the item is associated with **(A) only**
B if the item is associated with **(B) only**
C if the item is associated with **both (A) and (B)**
D if the item is associated with **neither (A) nor (B)**

Questions 122–126

For each characteristic listed below, select the disease with which it is most likely to be associated.

(A) Toxoplasmosis
(B) Histoplasmosis
(C) Both
(D) Neither

122. It is caused by a small yeast

123. It is a protozoan infection

124. It causes cerebral calcification and retino-choroiditis

125. It is penicillin-sensitive

126. It is treated with pyrimethamine and sulfonamides

Questions 127–133

For each characteristic of a vitamin deficiency listed below, select the disease with which it is most likely to be associated.

(A) Pellagra
(B) Beriberi
(C) Both
(D) Neither

127. Results from a nicotinic acid (niacin) deficiency

128. Results from a thiamine hydrochloride (vitamin B_1) deficiency

129. Results from a riboflavin (vitamin B_2) deficiency

130. Presents with diarrhea and dermatitis

131. Progresses to degenerative changes in the central nervous system

132. Can present as Wernicke's encephalopathy

133. Can be associated with pernicious anemia

Questions 134–138

Match the following.

(A) Rods
(B) Cones
(C) Both
(D) Neither

134. Mainly responsible for scotopic vision

135. Located in the periphery of the retina

136. Involved in color vision

137. Is a light-sensitive receptor of the retina

138. Contains large quantities of rhodopsin

Questions 139–143

Match the following.

(A) Tetanus toxoid
(B) Tetanus antitoxin
(C) Both
(D) Neither

139. Prepared by chemical denaturation of active neurotoxin

140. If produced in an animal host and administered to man, may cause serum sickness

141. Produces antibody against tetanus bacteria

142. Produced by a host during active infection with *Clostridium tetani*

143. Is bactericidal

Questions 144–148

For each sign or symptom listed below, select the vitamin that is most likely to be deficient.

(A) Vitamin A
(B) Vitamin D
(C) Both
(D) Neither

144. Night-blindness

145. Xerophthalmia

146. Osteomalacia

147. Bone deformities

148. Prolonged prothrombin time

Directions: The groups of questions below consist of lettered choices followed by several numbered items. For each numbered item select the **one** lettered choice with which it is **most** closely associated. Each lettered choice may be used once, more than once, or not at all.

Questions 149–154

Each of the lettered curves in the figure below summarizes the relationship between the velocity of an enzyme-catalyzed reaction as a function of substrate concentration. For each of the situations listed below, select the lettered curve on the graph that is most likely to be associated with it.

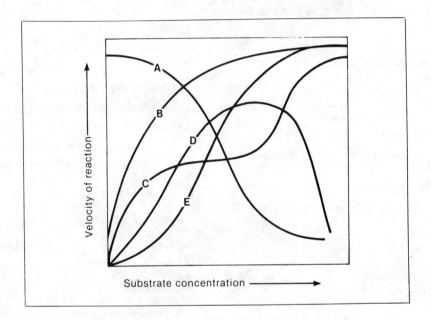

149. An enzyme-catalyzed reaction that obeys typical Michaelis-Menten kinetics

150. An enzyme that is inhibited by excess substrate

151. An enzyme exhibiting positive allosteric kinetics

152. If "enzyme activity" were substituted for "velocity of reaction" and "pH" were substituted for "substrate concentration," this curve would represent a typical pH-activity plot of an enzyme-catalyzed reaction

153. If "percent saturation of hemoglobin with oxygen" were substituted for "velocity of reaction" and "P_{O_2}" were substituted for "substrate concentration," this curve would represent an oxygen–hemoglobin dissociation curve

154. If "percent saturation of hemoglobin with oxygen" were substituted for "velocity of reaction" and "P_{O_2}" were substituted for "substrate concentration," this curve would represent an oxygen–myoglobin dissociation curve

Questions 155–159

For each of the drug effects listed below, select the antihypertensive medication most likely to cause it.

(A) Prazosin
(B) Trimethaphan
(C) Saralasin
(D) Triamterene
(E) Captopril

155. A nonaldosterone-dependent potassium-sparing medication

156. Inhibits formation of angiotensin II from angiotensin I

157. A ganglionic blocker used for controlled hypotension

158. An angiotensin II analogue

159. Selective postsynaptic α_1-adrenergic receptor antagonist

Questions 160–164

Study the diagram below, and then match the arteries or nerves listed below with the lettered structures in the diagram.

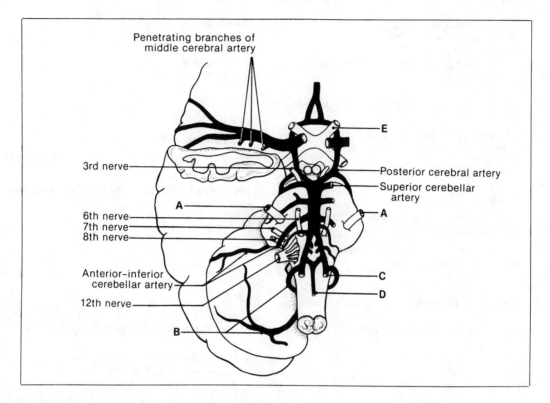

160. Trigeminal nerve

161. Posterior–inferior cerebellar artery

162. Vertebral artery

163. Anterior spinal artery

164. Third cranial nerve

Questions 165–169

Match each etiologic agent with the condition that it is most likely to cause.

(A) Gas gangrene
(B) Lockjaw
(C) Trench mouth
(D) Rice-water stools
(E) Blindness

165. *Clostridium novyi*

166. *Vibrio cholerae*

167. *Treponema vincentii*

168. *Chlamydia trachomatis*

169. *Clostridium tetani*

Questions 170–175

Match the following.

(A) Somatostatin
(B) Spironolactone
(C) Somatomedin
(D) Somatotropin
(E) Somesthetic cortex

170. Discrete localization of sensation

171. Growth hormone

172. Stimulated by growth hormone

173. Aldosterone antagonist

174. Growth hormone inhibitor

175. Produced by the anterior pituitary

Questions 176–181

For each description of cardiac function or location listed below, select the conduction pathway with which it is most likely to be associated.

(A) Atrioventricular node
(B) Sinoatrial node
(C) Purkinje system
(D) Arterial baroreceptors (pressoreceptors)
(E) None of the above

176. It is located in the posterior wall of the right atrium

177. Intrinsic depolarization rate is approximately 72/min

178. It is the normal "pacemaker" of the heart

179. Conduction velocity of the action potential is the fastest here

180. Conduction velocity of the excitatory process is exceedingly slow here

181. Frequency of firing is proportional to the hydrostatic pressure change

Questions 182–186

For each disease listed below, select the vitamin deficiency or toxicity with which it is most closely associated.

(A) Vitamin A
(B) Nicotinic acid
(C) Vitamin B_{12}
(D) Vitamin B_1
(E) Vitamin D_3

182. Pellagra

183. Beriberi

184. Pernicious anemia

185. Renal calculi and metastatic calcification of soft tissue

186. Tunnel vision and follicular hyperkeratosis

Questions 187–190

For each distribution curve listed below, select the diagram with which it is most closely associated.

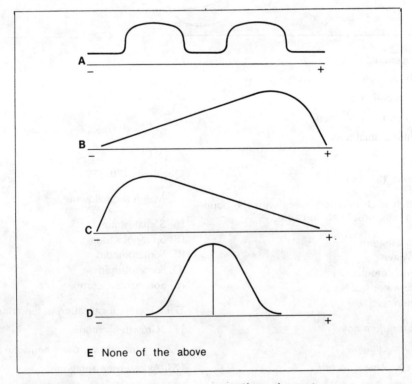

E None of the above

187. Normal distribution curve

188. Bimodal distribution curve

189. Skewed negative curve

190. Skewed positive curve

Questions 191–196

Match the following.

(A) Atropine
(B) Methacholine
(C) Physostigmine
(D) Succinylcholine
(E) Botulinum toxin

191. A parasympathetic (cholinergic) agonist

192. An anticholinesterase

193. A parasympathetic antagonist

194. A depolarizing neuromuscular blocking drug

195. Blocks acetylcholine release

196. A synonym for eserine

Questions 197–201

Match the following.

(A) Bromocriptine
(B) Danazol
(C) Clomiphene
(D) Metyrapone
(E) Methimazole

197. Blocks glucocorticoid synthesis

198. A dopamine agonist

199. Inhibitor of thyroid hormone synthesis

200. Suppresses gonadotropin secretion

201. An antiestrogenic agent

Questions 202–206

Match the letters in the photomicrograph below, which shows the layers of the retina, with the correct description of the layer.

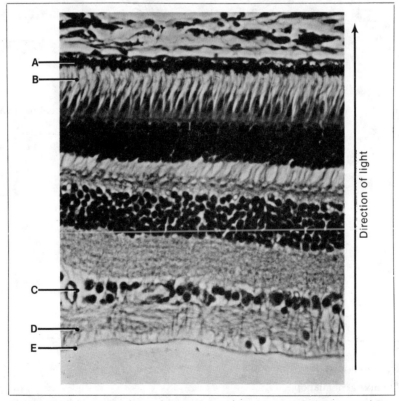

Reprinted with permission from Johnson KE: *Histology: Microscopic Anatomy and Embryology*. New York, John Wiley, 1982, p 385.

202. Pigmented epithelium

203. Rod and cone outer segments

204. Ganglion cell layer

205. Layer of optic nerve fibers

206. Inner limiting membrane

Questions 207–213

The diagram below illustrates a number of lesions specific to locations in the visual pathway. Match the optic defects listed below with the lesions in the visual fields in the figure.

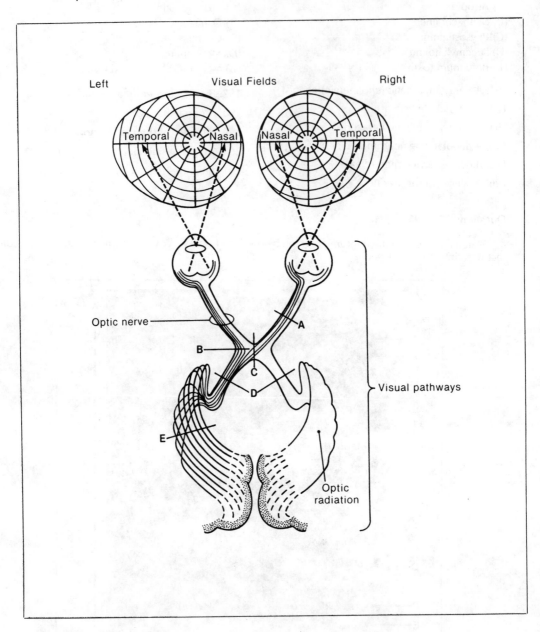

207. Right homonymous hemianopia

208. Bitemporal hemianopia

209. Glioma of the optic chiasm

210. Left nasal hemianopia

211. Total blindness in the right eye only

212. Total blindness

213. Craniopharyngioma can cause this lesion

Questions 214–218

For each definition listed below, select the term that it most accurately describes.

(A) Incidence
(B) Prevalence
(C) Mortality
(D) Morbidity
(E) Validity

214. True accuracy of observed experimental effects

215. Ratio of the number of ill persons to the total population of a community

216. Death rate in a given population

217. Rate of *all* cases of a phenomenon in a given population

218. Rate of *new* cases of a phenomenon in a given population

Questions 219–223

For each definition listed below, select the measure of dispersion that it most closely defines.

(A) Mean
(B) Mode
(C) Median
(D) Variance
(E) Range

219. Highest and lowest scores of a distribution

220. Standard deviation squared

221. Point above and below which 50% of all scores occur

222. Most frequent score

223. Arithmetic average of individual scores

Questions 224–228

For each untoward side effect listed below, select the drug most likely to be associated with it.

(A) Tamoxifen
(B) Streptozocin (streptozotocin)
(C) Cisplatin
(D) Ethambutol
(E) Methysergide

224. Retroperitoneal fibrosis

225. Retrobulbar neuritis

226. Ototoxicity and nephrotoxicity

227. Renal tubular damage

228. Hot flashes and bone pain

Questions 229–233

For each of the management protocols listed below, select the type of poisoning for which it would be most effective.

(A) Iron poisoning
(B) Arsenic poisoning
(C) Lead poisoning
(D) Salicylate poisoning
(E) Morphine sulphate overdose

229. Naloxone, 0.4–0.8 mg intravenously

230. Dimercaprol (BAL), plus antihistamine to reduce side effects of BAL

231. Calcium disodium edetate

232. Gastric lavage and alkalinization of the urine

233. Deferoxamine mesylate

Questions 234–239

For each drug effect listed below, select the antihypertensive agent most likely to cause it.

(A) Hydrochlorothiazide
(B) Hydralazine
(C) Reserpine
(D) Guanethidine
(E) Phenoxybenzamine

234. Blocks norepinephrine release from peripheral adrenergic nerves

235. Causes hyperuricemia

236. Releases insulin in pheochromocytoma

237. Results in impotence

238. Leads to neurotransmitter depletion

239. Confined to smooth muscle of arterioles

Questions 240–244

For each vitamin listed below, select the metabolic process with which it is most likely to be associated.

(A) Synthesis of amino acids
(B) Synthesis of DNA
(C) Calcium metabolism
(D) Oxidative phosphorylation
(E) Pentose phosphate pathway

240. Pyridoxal phosphate (vitamin B_6)

241. Folic acid (pteroylglutamic acid)

242. Cholecalciferol (vitamin D_3)

243. Niacin (nicotinic acid)

244. Thiamine (vitamin B_1)

Questions 245–250

Match each bone of the hand listed below with the correct letter on the x-ray.

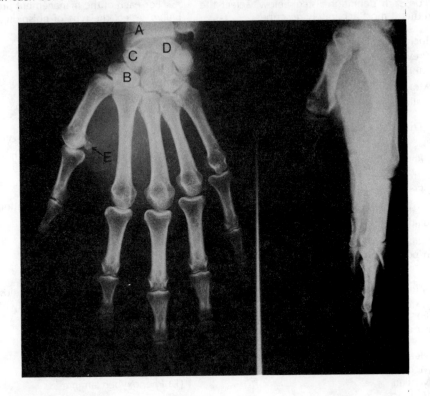

245. Trapezoid

246. Sesamoid

247. Lunate

248. Scaphoid

249. Distal end of the radius

250. Fracture of this bone is associated with avascular necrosis

Section B

Clinical Pharmacology
•
Medicine
•
Obstetrics and Gynecology
•
Pediatrics
•
Preventive Medicine and Public Health
•
Psychiatry
•
Surgery

Time—4 hours
Number of questions—250

QUESTIONS

Directions: Each question below contains five suggested answers. Choose the **one best** response to each question.

251. A physician is called because a patient has been given the wrong blood group, and she is very ill. The immunologic reaction to be expected in this situation is

(A) chronic rejection
(B) acute or accelerated reaction
(C) hyperacute reaction
(D) graft rejection of host
(E) none of the above

252. Effective prophylaxis against meningococcal meningitis is

(A) ampicillin, 3.5 g orally immediately
(B) meningococcal, serogroups A and C, polysaccharide vaccines
(C) sulfadiazine, 0.5 g four times a day for 5 days
(D) rifampin, 600 mg twice daily for 2 days
(E) not presently available

253. A young man presents with the scalp problem pictured below. There is no history of baldness in the family. He has not suffered any physical or chemical trauma to the scalp. He has also not taken any medications. Microscopic examination of scrapings from the scalp and mounted in potassium hydroxide revealed no abnormalities. The diagnosis is

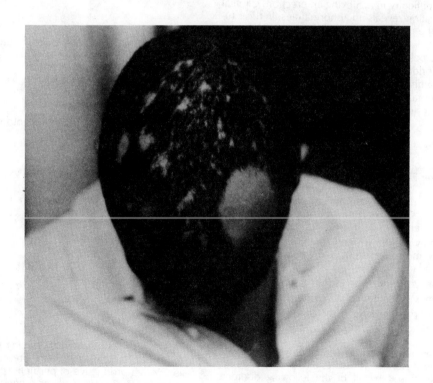

(A) male pattern baldness
(B) alopecia areata
(C) trichotillomania
(D) tinea capitis
(E) adrenogenital syndrome

254. Coarctation of the aorta is a congenital constriction usually distal to the ligamentum arteriosum. In a patient with such a lesion, the blood pressure readings will be

(A) unequal in both arms
(B) higher in the arms than the legs
(C) higher in the legs than the arms
(D) equal in the upper and lower extremities
(E) higher in the right arm and leg than in the left arm and leg

255. Platelet function is measured by

(A) prothrombin time
(B) bleeding time
(C) partial thromboplastin time
(D) platelet count
(E) removing fibrinogen from plasma

256. An anxious 24-year-old man presents with premature ejaculation, although he reports having no difficulty in achieving an erection. Clinical examination reveals no abnormalities. In this situation, the physician could prescribe

(A) metoclopramide
(B) thioridazine
(C) vitamin E
(D) propranolol
(E) testosterone

257. All of the following statements about the Zollinger-Ellison syndrome are true EXCEPT

(A) it is due to gastrinomas (non-β islet cell tumors) that occur in the pancreas and the duodenum
(B) it may present with epigastric pain that is usually more persistent and less responsive to standard ulcer therapy
(C) it may present with diarrhea
(D) it may present with steatorrhea
(E) most patients have resectable lesions

258. The adrenogenital syndrome, which is associated with elevated 17-ketosteroids and testosterone, can be caused by all of the following disorders EXCEPT

(A) congenital adrenal hyperplasia
(B) "postpubertal" adrenal hyperplasia
(C) Cushing's syndrome
(D) adrenal adenoma
(E) adrenal carcinoma

259. Remission of hyperglycemia is not infrequent in type II (noninsulin-dependent) diabetes mellitus and may be due to all of the following EXCEPT

(A) caloric restriction or weight reduction
(B) stopping thiazide diuretics
(C) reducing stress
(D) taking prednisolone
(E) increasing physical activity

260. A 1-month-old infant is brought into the physician's consulting room with a history of vomiting that has become progressively worse and is now "projectile." The vomitus is not bile stained. The infant is constipated, and the mother says that the infant's stools "resemble the fecal pellets of a rabbit." The most likely diagnosis in this infant is

(A) duodenal atresia
(B) acholuric jaundice
(C) cholecystitis
(D) pyloric stenosis
(E) volvulus neonatorum

261. Myasthenia gravis is a chronic autoimmune disease that is characterized by all of the following signs and symptoms EXCEPT

(A) muscle weakness
(B) absence of a thymus
(C) depletion of acetylcholine receptors
(D) fatigability
(E) presence of antibodies

262. All of the following conditions are associated with hypokalemia EXCEPT

(A) chronic diarrhea
(B) villous adenoma
(C) primary (hyper) aldosteronism
(D) hyperparathyroidism
(E) Cushing's syndrome

263. The x-rays shown on the facing page were taken of a middle-aged man presenting with fever, cough productive of purulent sputum, and chest pain. Radiologic findings suggest

(A) aspergillosis
(B) pericardial effusion
(C) right middle lobe pneumonia
(D) active tuberculosis
(E) none of the above

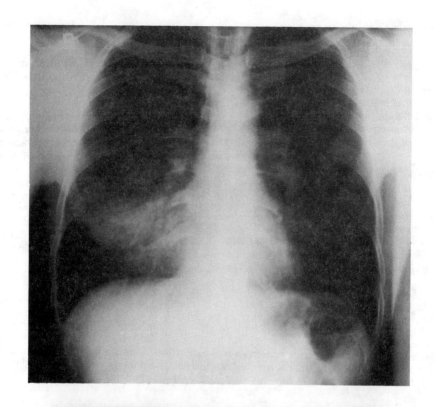

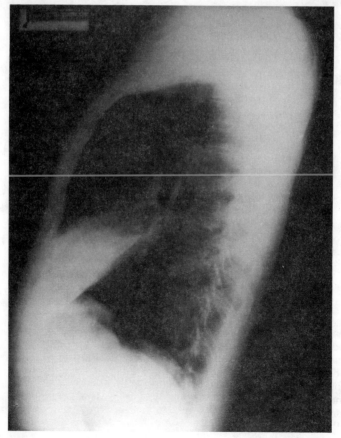

264. A neonate repeatedly vomits bile-stained fluid. Radiologic examination of the abdomen shows a "double-bubble" sign. The most likely diagnosis is

(A) meconium ileus
(B) duodenal atresia
(C) Meckel's diverticulum
(D) Hirschsprung's disease
(E) none of the above

265. Serum alkaline phosphatase may be elevated in all of the following individuals EXCEPT

(A) children
(B) pregnant women
(C) individuals with cholangiolar obstruction
(D) individuals with hypothyroidism
(E) individuals with osteoblastic bone disease

266. Which of the following statements concerning maternal mortality is true?

(A) Maternal mortality is higher from childbearing than it is from legal abortion, sterilization, and temporary methods of contraception combined
(B) Maternal mortality from all causes has been increasing slowly since the early 1970s
(C) Maternal mortality rates by race reveal approximately equal rates for white and black women
(D) Maternal mortality rates by age reveal approximately equal rates for all women in their reproductive years
(E) With the advent of ultrasound and other sophisticated diagnostic procedures, ectopic pregnancy is no longer considered a major cause of maternal mortality

267. The young woman in the photograph below is planning to get married soon and wants the cosmetically embarrassing swelling in her neck to be removed. Clinical examination and blood tests indicate that she is euthyroid; thyroid antimicrosomal autoantibodies are absent. The swelling is not tender and moves freely with swallowing. No bruits are audible. No associated lymphadenopathy is present, and there is no evidence of retrosternal extension. Ophthalmologic examination is normal. There is no family history of any endocrine disorder. She is not taking any pills (including contraceptives). Which of the following statements is applicable to this patient?

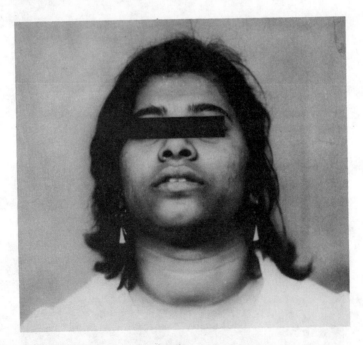

(A) The patient should be told to reduce her intake of iodized salt
(B) Radiotherapy may be useful to shrink the size of the swelling
(C) Propylthiouracil is useful but should be given for 3 months only
(D) Surgery is contraindicated
(E) None of the above

268. A 32-year-old man on clinical examination has tremors in both arms and his face. He is restless and agitated. He is sweating and has tachycardia and dilated pupils. He has been hearing voices for the past 10 days. The most likely diagnosis is

(A) brain tumor
(B) viral encephalitis
(C) pheochromocytoma
(D) delirium tremens
(E) tardive dyskinesia

269. All of the following statements regarding mammography done with specialized equipment are true EXCEPT

(A) it is the most effective diagnostic technique to detect nonpalpable or minimal breast cancer
(B) it may not reveal medullary carcinoma of the breast
(C) annual mammograms are recommended for all women over 40 years of age
(D) for every rad of radiation, six new cases of carcinoma of the breast per million women will be detected after a 10-year latent period
(E) if carcinoma of the breast is diagnosed by a competent radiologist, a biopsy is not necessary

270. All of the following statements regarding osteogenic sarcoma are true EXCEPT

(A) osteogenic sarcoma is the second most common (after plasma cell myeloma) primary malignant tumor of the bone
(B) 90% of the cases of primary osteogenic sarcoma involve the appendicular skeleton
(C) if left untreated, osteogenic sarcoma will metastasize most frequently to the lung, leading to an early death
(D) periosteal reaction, giving rise to "Codman's triangle" radiologically, is pathognomonic
(E) although it can occur at any age, osteogenic sarcoma is predominantly a disease of young men

271. Topical 5-fluorouracil cream may be effective in treatment of

(A) rodent ulcer
(B) Bowen's disease
(C) tinea versicolor
(D) solar keratosis
(E) pityriasis rosea

Questions 272 and 273

A 9-month-old infant is brought to the emergency room screaming. The mother says that the child has been experiencing paroxysms of abdominal colic with screaming and turning pale over the past 8–10 hours. The child has been well prior to this. The mother has also noticed a slimy, bloody discharge from the rectum. After sedating the child, clinical examination reveals a sausage-shaped mass in the left upper quadrant of the abdomen. Gentle rectal examination reveals red "currant jelly" stools.

272. The most likely diagnosis is

(A) Hirschsprung's disease
(B) intussusception
(C) meconium ileus
(D) pyloric stenosis
(E) volvulus neonatorum

273. After assessing this patient, one of the following procedures is undertaken and the child is cured. Which procedure is most likely to be performed?

(A) Urgent sigmoidoscopy
(B) Urgent barium meal
(C) Urgent and careful barium enema
(D) Urgent laparotomy
(E) Colostomy

(end of group question)

274. All of the following factors predispose to rupture of the uterus during labor EXCEPT

(A) cephalopelvic disproportion
(B) previous cesarean section
(C) advanced maternal age
(D) multiparity
(E) hypotonic uterine inertia

275. Exposure to asbestos may be causally associated with all of the following conditions EXCEPT

(A) mesothelioma
(B) pleural plaques
(C) bronchogenic carcinoma
(D) nasal septal ulceration
(E) pulmonary interstitial fibrosis

276. The man in the photograph below was asked to close his eyes and smile. He is most likely to be suffering from

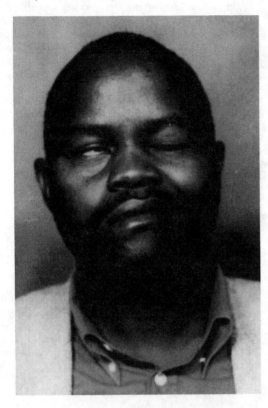

(A) paralysis agitans
(B) Huntington's chorea
(C) Bell's palsy
(D) a lesion of the eighth cranial nerve
(E) myasthenia gravis

277. Baseline mammography and physical examination are indicated in

(A) women between 35–40 years of age or older
(B) women with a mother or sister with premenopausal breast cancer
(C) women with endometrial cancer
(D) women with a breast cyst
(E) all of the above women

278. All of the following drugs are icterogenic as a result of hepatocellular toxicity EXCEPT

(A) halothane
(B) chlorpromazine
(C) phenobarbital
(D) oral contraceptives
(E) isoniazid

279. A 24-year-old law student is brought into the emergency room complaining of severe abdominal pain of 6–8 hours duration. He had been to a party the night before. The pain is in the epigastrium radiating to the back and is associated with nausea. The patient vomited twice prior to coming to the emergency room. Clinical examination reveals an anxious, acutely ill youth with a regular pulse rate of 100/min, blood pressure of 100/68 mm Hg, and a temperature of 38.1°C. The most likely diagnosis is

(A) acute appendicitis
(B) acute cholecystitis
(C) acute diverticulitis
(D) acute pancreatitis
(E) mesenteric adenitis

280. Which of the following statements about Paget's disease of the bone (osteitis deformans) is correct?

(A) Nerve deafness is a recognized feature
(B) The long bones are characteristically spared
(C) Hypercalcemia is usually present
(D) Alkaline phosphatase is usually normal
(E) Blue discoloration of the sclerae is pathognomonic

Questions 281 and 282

A 14-year-old boy complains of sore throat, fever, and cervical lymphadenopathy. The Paul-Bunnell test is positive.

281. The etiologic agent is

(A) cytomegalovirus
(B) gram-positive bacilli
(C) acid-fast bacilli
(D) Australian antigen
(E) Epstein-Barr virus

282. The above patient develops acute abdominal pain on the tenth day of his illness, and while the physician examines his abdomen, he suddenly becomes cold, pale, and sweaty with a rapid pulse. The physician should treat this patient with which of the following regimens?

(A) Immediate laparotomy
(B) Central venous pressure line, intravenous fluids, and observation
(C) Immediate intravenous pyelogram and intravenous antispasmodics
(D) Urgent gastroscopy
(E) None of the above regimens

(end of group question)

283. All of the following clinical presentations are typical of individuals with Plummer-Vinson syndrome EXCEPT

(A) dysphagia
(B) koilonychia
(C) glossitis
(D) fatigue
(E) raised hemosiderin in bone marrow

284. Classic hemophilia (factor VIII deficiency) is characterized by all of the following statements EXCEPT

(A) it is associated with a normal bleeding time (except after aspirin ingestion)
(B) it is associated with a positive family history in 90% of cases
(C) although the gene for factor VIII is on the X chromosome, the disease is manifested in men
(D) it is associated with a normal prothrombin time
(E) it can be successfully treated by infusion of banked plasma

285. Hypercalcemia may be caused by

(A) acute pancreatitis
(B) magnesium deficiency
(C) sarcoidosis
(D) pseudohypoparathyroidism
(E) hyperphosphatemia

286. A classic presentation of Alzheimer's disease includes all of the following EXCEPT

(A) it does not have a characteristic symptom complex
(B) it is associated with a Kayser-Fleischer ring in the eyes of most patients
(C) it usually develops insidiously
(D) it may begin with the amnesic syndrome
(E) it may present with dementia accompanied by delirium, delusions, or depression

287. African sleeping sickness may have all of the following clinical features EXCEPT

(A) a positive serologic test for syphilis
(B) fever, tachycardia, splenomegaly, and lymphadenopathy
(C) an inflammatory reaction at the site of inoculation
(D) trypanosomes in the cerebrospinal fluid in the late stage
(E) periorbital edema and barrel-shaped eggs in stools

288. An anxious, intelligent, and very religious 35-year-old woman with four children comes to her physician for some advice. She does not want to conceive again as her youngest child is only 1 year old, and her husband has just lost his job. Their religion forbids any form of artificial birth control. She menstruates regularly every 34 days for 4 days. The physician should tell her that she is most likely to ovulate on

(A) day 10 of her cycle
(B) day 15 of her cycle
(C) day 20 of her cycle
(D) day 25 of her cycle
(E) none of the above

289. All of the following statements about ectopic pregnancy are true EXCEPT

(A) ectopic pregnancy is more common in white women than in nonwhite women
(B) the fallopian tube is the most common site of ectopic nidation
(C) women with an intrauterine contraceptive device have a 10 times greater chance of ectopic pregnancy than other women
(D) vaginal examination may reveal exquisite tenderness
(E) Cullen's sign is a rare finding

290. The "extrinsic system" of the coagulation cascade is measured mainly by

(A) prothrombin time
(B) partial thromboplastin time
(C) bleeding time
(D) fibrinogen assay
(E) none of the above

291. Cushing's syndrome is characterized by all of the following EXCEPT

(A) centripetal obesity
(B) depression
(C) impaired glucose tolerance
(D) muscle hypertrophy
(E) osteoporosis

292. Women with a higher than normal risk of developing breast cancer include all of the following EXCEPT those who

(A) have a first-degree relative who has been treated for breast cancer
(B) have endometrial carcinoma
(C) are nulliparous
(D) have their first full-term pregnancy after 35 years of age
(E) use exogenous estrogens for menopausal symptoms

293. Herpes simplex virus type 1 (HSV-1) has which of the following characteristics?

(A) It is an RNA virus
(B) It is not associated with genital herpes infections
(C) The incubation period is 4–6 weeks
(D) It usually presents with a painful balanitis
(E) After the primary infection, a latent infection develops in the trigeminal ganglion

294. The first words that an infant speaks are

(A) adjectives
(B) verbs
(C) pronouns
(D) proverbs
(E) nouns

295. Congenital toxoplasmosis in the neonate is characterized by all of the following signs EXCEPT

(A) microcephaly
(B) convulsions
(C) mental retardation
(D) chorioretinitis
(E) bullous eruptions on the palms and soles

296. A middle-aged man presents with a mass on the left side of the neck. This mass is painless and mobile from side to side but not vertically. No bruit is audible over the mass. The most likely diagnosis is

(A) carotid body tumor
(B) carotid artery aneurysm
(C) tuberculous cervical lymphadenopathy
(D) cystic hygroma
(E) thyroglossal cyst

297. Herpes simplex virus type 2 (HSV-2) has all of the following characteristics EXCEPT

(A) it is usually acquired during childhood
(B) latent infections can be triggered by menstruation or anxiety
(C) recurrent episodes are usually less severe than the primary infection
(D) no vaccine is yet available for primary prevention
(E) there is some cross-immunity between HSV-1 and HSV-2 that confers partial protection with the heterologous virus

298. Fertilization of the ovum usually occurs in

(A) the cornu uteri
(B) the outer one-third of the fallopian tube
(C) the corpus uteri
(D) the cervical canal
(E) none of the above

Questions 299–301

A 32-year-old woman presents with a cough productive of mucopurulent sputum. She also complains of paresthesias, constipation, and a gritty feeling in her eyes. Clinical examination reveals nothing remarkable except slight conjunctival congestion, bilateral rhonchi, and a nonspecific rash on her neck and the dorsum of her left hand. Microscopy of sputum is negative for acid-fast bacilli, and culture of sputum for bacteria and fungi yields no growth. Tuberculin testing shows no reaction.

299. The x-rays on the facing page suggest which of the following diagnoses?

(A) Tuberculosis
(B) Rheumatoid arthritis
(C) Aspergillosis
(D) Carcinoma of the bronchus
(E) Sarcoidosis

300. Which of the following findings would be most useful in substantiating the diagnosis?

(A) Elevated erythrocyte sedimentation rate
(B) Negative culture for *Mycobacterium tuberculosis* after 1 month
(C) Negative rheumatoid complement fixation test
(D) Normal serum protein levels and a serum calcium of 11.2 mg/dl
(E) High titers of immunoglobulin E

301. The electrocardiogram done on this patient is likely to reveal

(A) large peaked T waves
(B) prominent U waves
(C) prolonged QRS complex
(D) shortened QT interval
(E) none of the above

(end of group question)

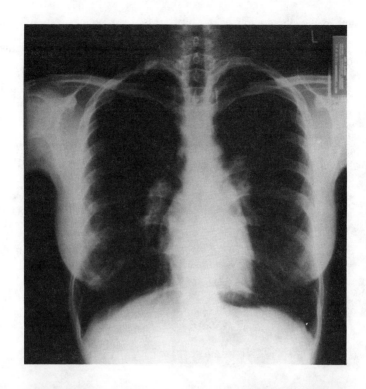

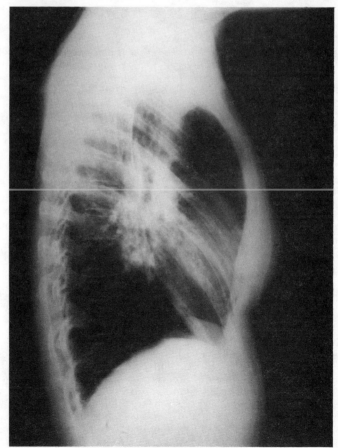

302. The patient in the photograph below presents with a lesion on the right side of his face that is discharging pus containing sulfur granules. This is most likely due to

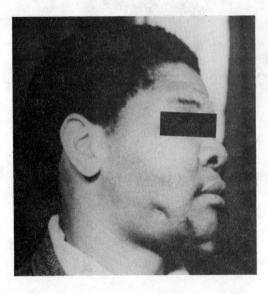

(A) a fungal infection
(B) a viral infection
(C) an anaerobic bacterial infection
(D) a rickettsial infection
(E) none of the above

303. Down's syndrome has all of the following clinical features EXCEPT

(A) mental retardation
(B) Brushfield's spots
(C) muscular hypotonicity
(D) "setting sun" sign of eyes
(E) short, curved little fingers due to a hypoplastic middle phalanx

Questions 304 and 305

A 22-year-old emaciated man presents to a physician in a remote village in a tsetse fly–infested area in Africa. He complains of night sweats, weight loss, lethargy, and financial embarrassment. On examination, he is found to have a distended abdomen, but there is no evidence of intestinal obstruction. No special investigations are available except for urinalysis, which reveals a slight hematuria, and an erythrocyte sedimentation rate (ESR) done by the Westergren method, which is markedly elevated.

304. The physician should give the patient

(A) instructions to go to the nearest teaching hospital, which is 600 miles away, and the only form of transport is a horse-drawn cart
(B) 1.5 g ampicillin intravenously every 6 hr
(C) intravenous vitamins and restrict salt intake
(D) streptomycin, isoniazid, and ethambutol in combination
(E) 1.0 g metronidazole every 6 hr

305. After adopting one of the above suggestions, the patient appears to improve but he tells you that he cannot see the color green, especially with the right eye. Thus, the physician should do which of the following?

(A) Administer large doses of vitamin A
(B) Administer digoxin
(C) Stop ethambutol
(D) Stop metronidazole
(E) Administer pyridoxine

(end of group question)

306. The average breast x-ray dose for a routine two-view bilateral mammogram should ideally not exceed

(A) 1 rad
(B) 5 rad
(C) 10 rad
(D) 50 rad
(E) 100 rad

307. Mental retardation is associated with which of the following conditions?

(A) Maple syrup urine disease
(B) Cystinuria
(C) Alkaptonuria
(D) Acute intermittent porphyria
(E) Idiopathic lactase deficiency

308. Hyperkalemia may result from

(A) amphotericin B
(B) blood that has been stored for 14 days
(C) thiazide diuretics
(D) excessive licorice consumption
(E) carbenicillin

309. A young woman who has a 2-year-old child presents in the emergency room with acute pain in the right iliac fossa. She appears shocked with pallor, a thready pulse of 100/min, and blood pressure of 100/60 mm Hg. About 18 months ago she had an intrauterine device (IUD) inserted; she has had no problems with the IUD during this time. She is not aware of having missed a period; however, her periods have always been irregular, and, in any case, she started bleeding this morning. The most likely diagnosis is

(A) acute appendicitis
(B) Meckel's diverticulitis
(C) acute salpingitis
(D) Crohn's disease
(E) ectopic pregnancy

310. Although hyperbaric oxygen therapy may be beneficial in the management of all of the conditions listed below, it is most likely to cause complications in

(A) air embolism
(B) burns
(C) carbon monoxide poisoning
(D) gas gangrene
(E) hyaline membrane disease

311. The 9-year-old boy in the photograph below presents with a pruritic vesicular eruption. His mother says that the child has been feverish, "off color," and not eating well for the past 2 weeks. Scrapings taken from the base of one of the lesions show multinucleated giant cells with intranuclear inclusions. The diagnosis is

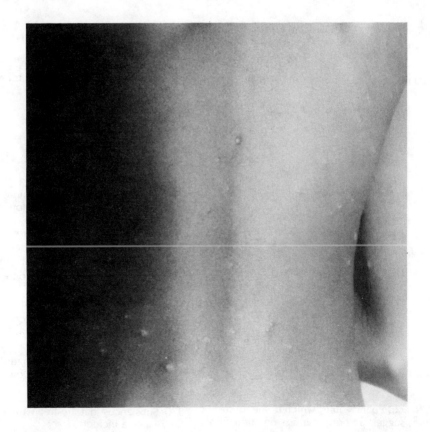

(A) chickenpox
(B) herpes zoster
(C) scabies
(D) syphilis
(E) none of the above

312. The "intrinsic pathway" of the coagulation cascade is measured by

(A) prothrombin time
(B) bleeding time
(C) partial thromboplastin time
(D) fibrinogen assay
(E) fibrinogen degradation products assay

313. Acanthosis nigricans may be associated with all of the following conditions EXCEPT

(A) gastric adenocarcinomas in the elderly
(B) melasma gravidarum
(C) Addison's disease
(D) diabetes mellitus
(E) Stein-Leventhal syndrome

314. The most common site of carcinoma in women is the

(A) breast
(B) cervix
(C) ovary
(D) uterus
(E) vagina

315. The fetal alcohol syndrome, resulting from maternal alcohol abuse, has all of the following clinical features EXCEPT

(A) microcephaly
(B) deafness
(C) low birth weight
(D) flattened facial features
(E) mild to moderate mental retardation

316. All of the following statements about pityriasis rosea are true EXCEPT it

(A) is due to a fungal infection
(B) is more commonly seen in women
(C) is usually preceded by a "herald patch"
(D) may be mistaken for secondary syphilis
(E) usually resolves completely in 6–8 weeks without treatment

Directions: Each question below contains four suggested answers of which **one or more** is correct. Choose the answer

A if **1, 2, and 3** are correct
B if **1 and 3** are correct
C if **2 and 4** are correct
D if **4** is correct
E if **1, 2, 3, and 4** are correct

317. Melasma may be due to

(1) syphilis
(2) pregnancy
(3) gold injections
(4) estrogens and progesterones

318. In acute pancreatitis, which of the following features suggest a poor prognosis on admission?

(1) Hypocalcemia (<8 mg/dl)
(2) Hyperglycemia (>200 mg/dl)
(3) Serum lactic dehydrogenase (>350 U/ml)
(4) Serum amylase (>3000 U/dl)

319. Correct statements concerning Down's syndrome include which of the following?

(1) Ninety-five percent of cases are due to trisomy 21, and five percent are due to translocations of chromosomes 21 and 22
(2) Children with Down's syndrome have an incidence of leukemia that is 15 times greater than the normal population
(3) Advanced paternal age accounts for about 25% of cases of Down's syndrome (trisomy 21)
(4) Physical examination distinguishes between trisomy and translocation Down's syndrome

320. Substances that are freely transferred across the placenta include

(1) IgG
(2) IgM
(3) warfarin
(4) IgA

321. Overdosage or prolonged administration of steroidal anti-inflammatory agents may exaggerate some of the normal physiologic actions of both mineralocorticoids and glucocorticoids and lead to deleterious effects, such as

(1) diabetes mellitus
(2) osteoporosis, resulting in vertebral collapse
(3) hypokalemic alkalosis
(4) progression of bacterial and fungal infections

322. Hashimoto's thyroiditis is a chronic autoimmune inflammation of the thyroid gland with which of the following features?

(1) It affects mainly men between the ages of 30 and 50 years
(2) Histologic examination reveals a lymphocyte and plasma cell infiltrate with varying amounts of fibrosis and the disappearance of thyroidal colloid
(3) As the disease progresses, hyperthyroidism associated with elevated levels of T_3 and T_4 develops
(4) Antibody to thyroid microsomal antigen can be detected by the complement fixation test

323. Raised serum iron is characteristically associated with which of the following conditions?

(1) Hemochromatosis
(2) Sideroblastic anemia
(3) Polycythemia vera
(4) Plummer-Vinson syndrome

324. Pseudogout is characterized by which of the following statements?

(1) It responds immediately to colchicine (4 mg) administered intramuscularly
(2) Crystals that exhibit weakly positive birefringence are diagnostic
(3) It accounts for 50% of all cases of calcium pyrophosphate dihydrate deposition disease
(4) It can cause fever and leukocytosis

325. Delirium may present with

(1) clouding of consciousness
(2) perceptual disturbances (e.g., hallucinations)
(3) disorientation
(4) memory impairment

326. A middle-aged man presents with a fungating mass on the sole of his foot pictured below. The mass initially began as a dark, pigmented growth. The physician should immediately manage this patient with

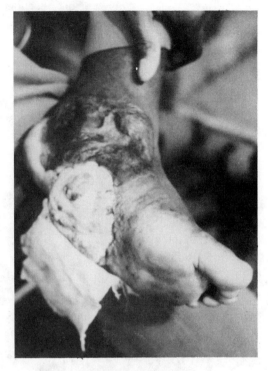

(1) cancer chemotherapy
(2) biopsy
(3) amputation
(4) radiologic examination

327. Acute intermittent porphyria may be precipitated by administration of which of the following drugs to a susceptible person?

(1) Estrogens
(2) Barbiturates
(3) Sulfonamides
(4) Griseofulvin

328. Low birth weight infants are commonly born to women who

(1) smoke more than 10 cigarettes a day
(2) are over 40 years of age
(3) are younger than 16 years of age
(4) are of low socioeconomic status

SUMMARY OF DIRECTIONS

A	B	C	D	E
1, 2, 3 only	1, 3 only	2, 4 only	4 only	All are correct

329. Tetralogy of Fallot, which is usually diagnosed in infancy and early childhood, consists of which of the following defects?

(1) Right ventricular hypertrophy
(2) Overriding aorta
(3) Ventricular septal defect
(4) Pulmonary valve stenosis

330. The 30-year-old patient in the photograph below presents with inadequate sexual performance (impotence). His speaking voice sounds like a young boy. The clinical findings likely to be observed in this patient include which of the following?

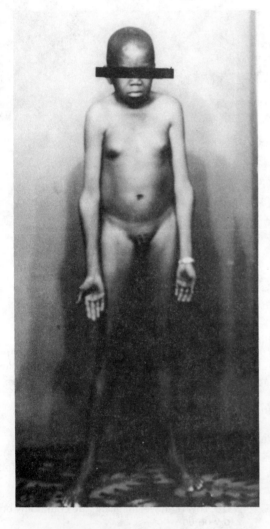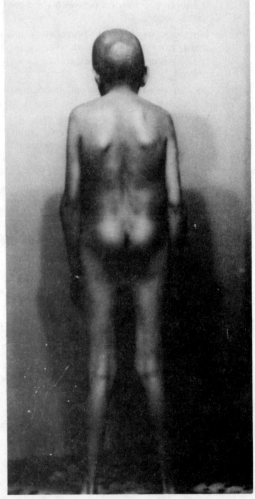

(1) A 47,XXY karyotype
(2) Turner's syndrome
(3) Leydig cell hyperplasia
(4) Normal sperm production

331. Gastric carcinoma has which of the following features?

(1) It is decreasing in incidence in the United States
(2) It usually appears at age 50 years or after
(3) Surgery is curative if it is detected early
(4) Carcinomatous ulcers can be distinguished from benign ulcers on gastroscopy

332. Giardiasis may be treated with

(1) quinacrine
(2) metronidazole
(3) furazolidone
(4) mepacrine

333. Disseminated intravascular coagulopathy may complicate

(1) abruptio placentae
(2) amniotic fluid embolism
(3) thrombotic thrombocytopenic purpura
(4) widespread carcinomatosis

334. Oral and genital lesions characteristically coexist in

(1) lymphogranuloma venereum
(2) Behçet's disease
(3) pityriasis rosea
(4) erythema multiforme

335. Petechiae are a recognized feature of

(1) neonatal hypoglycemia
(2) vitamin D deficiency
(3) acute rheumatic fever
(4) thrombocytopenia

336. Complications of electroconvulsive therapy include

(1) death
(2) memory disturbance
(3) respiratory arrest
(4) cardiac arrest

337. Correct statements concerning rabies infection include which of the following?

(1) It can cause hydrophobia
(2) It can have an incubation period of 1 year or more
(3) It can cause an encephalomyelitis
(4) It is caused by a DNA virus

338. Iron deficiency anemia is common in

(1) infants
(2) men
(3) menstruating women
(4) postmenopausal women

339. A physician is likely to come to which of the following conclusions concerning the condition of the patient in the photograph below?

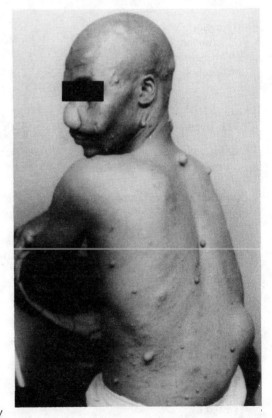

(1) It may be associated with deafness
(2) It may be associated with secondary hypertension
(3) It is associated with Lisch nodules in the iris
(4) It is inherited as an autosomal recessive trait

---

340. Giant "a" waves in the jugular venous pulse may be caused by

(1) atrial fibrillation
(2) tricuspid stenosis
(3) constrictive pericarditis
(4) severe cor pulmonale

341. Substances that are established teratogens include

(1) cyclophosphamide
(2) busulfan
(3) thalidomide
(4) alcohol

342. Hyperamylasemia may be associated with

(1) acute pancreatitis
(2) perforated peptic ulcer
(3) mumps
(4) the administration of narcotics

343. Lymphatic drainage of the breast includes drainage to the

(1) axillary nodes
(2) rectus sheath
(3) supraclavicular nodes
(4) internal thoracic nodes

344. Alcoholism (alcohol dependence) is suggested by

(1) the occurrence of blackouts
(2) early morning drinking
(3) sobriety in the presence of elevated alcohol levels
(4) solitary drinking

345. Congenital dislocation of the hip has which of the following characteristics?

(1) It occurs more frequently in boys
(2) It may not be recognized until the age of 1 year
(3) Surgery is the treatment of choice
(4) It is usually a unilateral deformity

346. Hyperbaric oxygen therapy is indicated in

(1) carbon monoxide poisoning
(2) decompression sickness
(3) air embolism
(4) gas gangrene

347. Early treatment in infancy may prevent mental retardation in which of the following diseases?

(1) Phenylketonuria
(2) Down's syndrome
(3) Cretinism
(4) Tay-Sachs disease

348. The pickwickian syndrome is characterized by

(1) nocturnal alveolar hypoventilation
(2) obesity
(3) daytime somnolence
(4) hypocapnia

349. Vitamin K is essential for the synthesis in the liver of which of the following factors?

(1) Prothrombin (factor II)
(2) Proconvertin (factor VII)
(3) Christmas factor (factor IX)
(4) Stuart factor (factor X)

350. Characteristics of an abused or neglected child include

(1) fatigue and retarded physical growth
(2) pseudomature behavior
(3) unexplained physical injuries
(4) recent history of enuresis and nightmares

Questions 351 and 352

The patient in the photograph below presents with a painful vesicular rash on the right side of the chest and on the right arm.

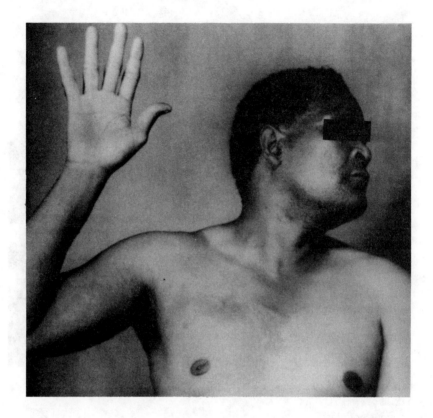

351. The pathogen responsible for the above condition has which of the following characteristics?

(1) It causes centripetal vesicular eruptions in children
(2) It is characterized by multinucleated giant cells with intranuclear inclusion bodies
(3) It is a DNA virus
(4) The course of this eruption is shortened by varicella zoster immune globulin

352. The above condition is likely to be complicated by

(1) purpura fulminans
(2) Guillain-Barré syndrome
(3) aseptic meningitis
(4) blackwater fever

(end of group question)

353. Risk factors for successful suicide include

(1) age over 45 years
(2) widowed or divorced status
(3) unemployed status
(4) being a woman

354. Congenital adrenal hyperplasia is characterized by which of the following statements?

(1) It may be due to a lack of 21-hydroxylase
(2) It is best treated by adrenalectomy
(3) It causes ambiguous genitalia in female children
(4) It is characterized by subnormal production of adrenocorticotropic hormone

355. The patient pictured below may have

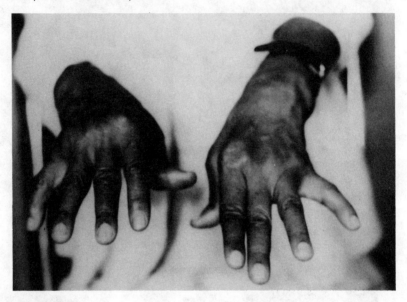

(1) antinuclear antibodies
(2) amyloidosis
(3) subcutaneous nodules
(4) hypogammaglobulinemia

356. The hypercalcemia that results from hyperparathyroidism in turn may cause

(1) short QT intervals
(2) anorexia
(3) psychosis
(4) hyperreflexia

357. The postphlebitic syndrome is characterized by

(1) edema, pain, and skin changes (i.e., eczema, induration, and pigmentation)
(2) ambulatory venous hypertension
(3) iliofemoral venous thrombosis
(4) insensitivity to fibrinolytic therapy

358. A patient in early pregnancy who is experiencing threatened abortion is likely to present with

(1) low gonadotropin levels and products of conception in the cervical canal
(2) vaginal bleeding or spotting
(3) ruptured membranes and mild abdominal cramps
(4) closed cervical os with mild abdominal cramps

359. Cauda equina neuropathy may present with

(1) sciatica
(2) brisk knee jerks
(3) disturbance in bladder function
(4) choreoathetosis

360. Raised serum iron is characteristically associated with

(1) thalassemia major
(2) pica
(3) sideroblastic anemia
(4) Plummer-Vinson syndrome

361. Which of the following conditions may be associated with secondary hyperuricemia?

(1) Lead poisoning
(2) Multiple myeloma
(3) Glucose 6-phosphate dehydrogenase deficiency
(4) Chronic renal failure

362. Marijuana intoxication characteristically presents with

(1) conjunctival injection
(2) distorted perception of time and space
(3) euphoria
(4) anorexia

363. Missed abortion can present with

(1) amenorrhea (for at least 2 months)
(2) malaise, anorexia, headache, and a peculiar taste in the mouth
(3) hypofibrinogenemia tendency
(4) high titer of chorionic gonadotropin

364. Characteristic features of tuberculoid leprosy include

(1) a positive lepromin skin test
(2) nodular skin lesions
(3) severe nerve involvement
(4) skin smears yielding abundant *Mycobacterium leprae*

365. Organic brain syndrome may be caused by

(1) uremia
(2) hepatic failure
(3) hypoglycemia
(4) diabetic ketoacidosis

366. The condition depicted in the picture below is

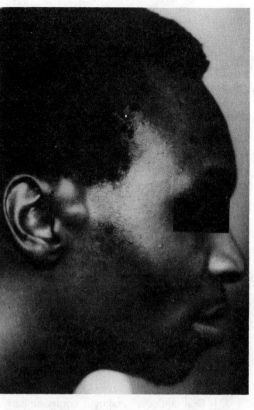

(1) due to fusion of the six tubercles that form the pinna
(2) due to tuberculosis
(3) treated surgically
(4) associated with congenital deafness

367. Recognized risk factors for cerebral thrombosis include which of the following?

(1) Polycythemia
(2) Thrombocytosis
(3) Oral contraceptives
(4) Heparin

368. Management of superficial venous thrombophlebitis includes

(1) elastic stockings or bandages
(2) strict bed rest
(3) administration of salicylates
(4) anticoagulation therapy

369. Conditions that are more common in women than men include

(1) primary biliary cirrhosis
(2) Sjögren's syndrome
(3) progressive systemic sclerosis
(4) systemic lupus erythematosus

370. Smoking may be a causal factor for which of the following conditions?

(1) Peptic ulcer disease
(2) Thromboangiitis obliterans
(3) Cancer of the urinary bladder
(4) Cancer of the esophagus

371. Oral cholecystography is contraindicated in the presence of which of the following conditions?

(1) Obstructive jaundice
(2) Gastroenteritis
(3) Severe hepatorenal disease
(4) Goiter

372. Recognized causes of neonatal jaundice include

(1) hypothyroidism
(2) breast-feeding associated with poor intake
(3) a large cephalhematoma
(4) the administration of phenobarbital

373. Delayed hypersensitivity plays a very important role in cell-mediated immunity and thus provides resistance to

(1) fungal infections
(2) viral infections
(3) tumors
(4) protozoal infections

374. Correct statements regarding deep vein thrombosis include which of the following?

(1) Venography is of no value in achieving a diagnosis
(2) Heparin must be started when the index of suspicion warrants it
(3) Elevation of the extremity is not effective
(4) Elastic stockings have no role in the acute phase of deep vein thrombosis but are valuable once the patient begins to walk

375. Possible responses in a patient suffering from digitalis toxicity include which of the following?

(1) Cardioversion may precipitate serious arrhythmias, such as ventricular tachycardia
(2) There may be ST segment changes, which usually occur as a depression from the baseline
(3) Propranolol may be helpful in treatment, provided there is no atrioventricular block
(4) Hallucinations and xanthopsia may occur

376. Postural hypotension may be due to

(1) diabetic neuropathy
(2) monoamine oxidase inhibitors
(3) prazosin
(4) dopamine

377. Hypothermia with a core temperature below 35°C may cause

(1) J waves on the electrocardiogram
(2) ventricular fibrillation
(3) hypoglycemia
(4) metabolic acidosis

378. Dementia classically presents with

(1) memory difficulties (especially recent memory)
(2) clouding of consciousness
(3) impaired judgment and emotional lability
(4) visual hallucinations

379. Chemotherapeutic drugs that are alkylating agents include which of the following?

(1) Mechlorethamine
(2) Cyclophosphamide
(3) Chlorambucil
(4) Methotrexate

380. Ankylosing spondylitis may be complicated by

(1) pulmonary fibrosis
(2) anterior uveitis
(3) aortic incompetence
(4) acute urethritis

381. Disseminated intravascular coagulopathy is characterized by

(1) thrombocytosis
(2) fibrinogenopenia
(3) absence of fibrin split products
(4) decreased factors V and VIII

382. The major circadian rhythms include which of the following?

(1) REM and non-REM variations in sleep
(2) Cell reproduction and sensitivity
(3) Sleep and wakefulness periods
(4) Menstrual cycles in women

383. Recognized features of untreated congenital pyloric stenosis include

(1) dehydration
(2) a raised plasma bicarbonate level
(3) an excess loss of potassium ion in the urine
(4) projectile vomiting

384. Complications of multiple myeloma include

(1) abnormal plasma cell infiltration of bone marrow
(2) amyloidosis
(3) raised serum calcium
(4) presence of the Philadelphia chromosome

385. Which of the following statements characterize hemifacial spasm?

(1) It can cause great physical and psychological distress
(2) Anticonvulsant drugs, such as phenytoin and carbamazepine, are usually effective
(3) It is more common in women
(4) It affects the right side more commonly than the left side

386. The Brown-Séquard syndrome results in

(1) disease on one side of the spinal cord
(2) loss of position and vibration sense
(3) contralateral loss of pain and temperature sensation
(4) contralateral spastic paralysis

387. Gout may be caused by

(1) thiazide diuretics
(2) cancer chemotherapy
(3) psoriasis
(4) overhydration

388. Parents reported for child abuse typically exhibit which of the following characteristics?

(1) They are neglectful of the child's physical hygiene
(2) They react excessively to the child's condition
(3) They are distrustful
(4) They are uncooperative

389. Manifestations of diabetic retinopathy include

(1) microaneurysms
(2) hard exudates
(3) hemorrhages
(4) proliferating new blood vessels

390. Neonatal goiter may be caused by

(1) ingestion of antithyroid drugs during pregnancy
(2) prolonged use of iodine-containing medicines during pregnancy
(3) an inborn error of metabolism
(4) maternal alcoholism

391. Goodpasture's syndrome is characterized by

(1) typical appearance of glomeruli on immunofluorescent staining
(2) cough and hemoptysis as presenting symptoms
(3) hypochromic iron deficiency anemia
(4) a good prognosis

SUMMARY OF DIRECTIONS

A	B	C	D	E
1, 2, 3 only	1, 3 only	2, 4 only	4 only	All are correct

392. Senile osteoporosis is characterized by

(1) pseudofracture
(2) low serum calcium
(3) high alkaline phosphatase activity
(4) a reduced number of bone trabeculae

393. Sudden peripheral arterial occlusion may present with

(1) pain
(2) pulselessness
(3) pallor
(4) shock

394. Complications of severe hypertension include

(1) encephalopathy
(2) congestive cardiac failure
(3) subarachnoid hemorrhage
(4) hyperglycemia

395. Correct statements about squamous cell carcinoma of the larynx include which of the following?

(1) It is found almost exclusively in smokers
(2) It predominates statistically in men, but the percentage of women with squamous cell carcinoma of the larynx appears to be increasing
(3) The combination of heavy smoking and heavy alcohol consumption increases the risk
(4) It affects approximately 9000 patients per year in the United States

396. Characteristics of cholelithiasis include which of the following?

(1) It is more common in diabetic individuals
(2) It is frequently asymptomatic
(3) It may be a predisposing factor in the development of gallbladder carcinoma
(4) It is more common in men between 30–80 years of age

397. Schizophrenia characteristically presents with

(1) disturbances in association
(2) disturbances in affect
(3) ambivalence
(4) autism

398. Reiter's syndrome is associated with

(1) nonspecific urethritis
(2) bamboo spine
(3) arthritis
(4) nephrolithiasis

399. Sarcoidosis may present with

(1) bilateral hilar lymphadenopathy and right paratracheal lymphadenopathy
(2) polyarthritis
(3) iridocyclitis
(4) pleural effusion

400. Electroconvulsive therapy is indicated for

(1) obsessive–compulsive neurosis
(2) hysteria
(3) delirium tremens
(4) major depression

401. Characteristics of erythrasma include which of the following?

(1) It most commonly affects toe webs
(2) Lesions are well-defined scaling plaques that resemble tinea versicolor or psoriasis
(3) It is diagnosed by a characteristic coral red fluorescence with Wood's light
(4) It is a fungal disease

402. Secondary pulmonary hypertension may be caused by

(1) kyphoscoliosis
(2) left ventricular failure
(3) mitral stenosis
(4) ventricular septal defect

403. Which of the following situations or substances may interfere with catecholamine determination in urine?

(1) Shock
(2) Ephedrine nose drops
(3) Methyldopa
(4) Thiazides and clonidine

404. Characteristics of Lyme arthritis include which of the following?

(1) It is caused by a spirochete
(2) The fluorescent treponemal antibody absorption test is positive
(3) It responds to tetracycline
(4) It is due to excess calcium deposits in the joints

405. Hemochromatosis is characterized by

(1) excessive saturation of transferrin
(2) pancreatic fibrosis and siderosis
(3) hemosiderin deposits in the liver
(4) low serum iron

Directions: The groups of questions below consist of lettered choices followed by several numbered items. For each numbered item, select the one lettered choice with which it is most closely associated. Each lettered choice may be used once, more than once, or not at all. Choose answer:

(A)   if the item is associated with **(A) only**
(B)   if the item is associated with **(B) only**
(C)   if the item is associated with **both (A) and (B)**
(D)   if the item is associated with **neither (A) nor (B)**

Questions 406–411

Match the following.

(A) Carbidopa
(B) Levodopa
(C) Both
(D) Neither

406. Passes the blood–brain barrier

407. Antiparkinsonian drug

408. Peripheral decarboxylase inhibitor

409. Converted to dopamine by dopa decarboxylase

410. Good urinary antiseptic

411. Effective antiviral drug

Questions 412–416

For each disease characteristic listed below, select the condition with which it is most closely associated.

(A) Delirium
(B) Schizophrenia
(C) Both
(D) Neither

412. Visual hallucinations are characteristic of this condition

413. Auditory hallucinations are characteristic of this condition

414. Lithium is the treatment of choice

415. Sudden withdrawal from barbiturates may precipitate this condition

416. It may be caused by hypoglycemia

Questions 417–420

For each of the statements below concerning effective treatment for gonorrhea or its complications, select the treatment of choice.

(A) Ampicillin
(B) Spectinomycin
(C) Both
(D) Neither

417. It can be used to treat gonorrhea if the patient is allergic to penicillin

418. A single injection is effective against penicillinase-producing *Neisseria gonorrhoeae*

419. It can be used to treat disseminated gonorrhea

420. It will prevent ophthalmia neonatorum if taken orally

Questions 421–426

For each characteristic listed below, select the disease with which it is most closely associated.

(A) Silicosis
(B) Asbestosis
(C) Both
(D) Neither

421. Gold miners and insulation manufacturing workers are predisposed to it

422. Shaver's disease is a common sequela

423. Pulmonary hypertension and cor pulmonale eventually develop

424. Lung infections, especially tuberculosis, are associated with it

425. "Eggshell" calcification of the lymph nodes is characteristic

426. A high incidence of malignant mesothelioma, even after trivial exposure, is associated with it

Questions 427–433

For each characteristic listed below, select the disease entity with which it is most likely to be associated.

(A) "Pink puffer"
(B) "Blue bloater"
(C) Both
(D) Neither

427. It is a manifestation of chronic obstructive pulmonary disease

428. Chest x-ray shows increased bronchovascular markings and cardiac enlargement

429. Sputum production is relatively scant

430. Residual lung volume is increased

431. Total lung capacity is normal or decreased

432. Blood studies usually show normal hematocrit, moderately reduced arterial oxygen saturation, and a low or normal carbon dioxide

433. Pulmonary hypertension and cor pulmonale are likely complications

Directions: The groups of questions below consist of lettered choices followed by several numbered items. For each numbered item select the **one** lettered choice with which it is **most** closely associated. Each lettered choice may be used once, more than once, or not at all.

Questions 434–438

For each animal or object listed below, select the disease for which a handler would be at risk.

(A) Sporotrichosis
(B) Psittacosis
(C) Anthrax
(D) Rabies
(E) Erysipeloid

434. Fish

435. Wild mammals

436. Hides

437. Birds

438. Decaying wood

Questions 439–443

Match the characteristics of the urogenital diseases listed below with the organism that is most likely to cause it.

(A) *Candida albicans*
(B) *Trichomonas vaginalis*
(C) *Gardnerella vaginalis*
(D) *Neisseria gonorrhoeae*
(E) Herpes simplex virus

439. It is associated with carcinoma of the cervix

440. It presents with pain in the right iliac fossa, and Gram stain of a cervical smear shows gram-negative diplococci

441. Greenish, frothy, vaginal discharge on wet-mount preparation shows motile flagellates on microscopy

442. It produces a "fishy" odor of vaginal discharge and "clue cells" on vaginal smear

443. It produces an irritating curdy vaginal discharge

Questions 444–451

For each untoward side effect listed below, select the chemotherapeutic agent most likely to be associated with it.

(A) Bleomycin
(B) Methotrexate
(C) Cyclophosphamide
(D) Vincristine
(E) Doxorubicin

444. Peripheral neuritis

445. Pulmonary fibrosis

446. Hemorrhagic cystitis

447. Cardiotoxicity

448. Sterility

449. Gastrointestinal ulceration

450. Syndrome of inappropriate diuretic hormone secretion

451. A folic acid antagonist and an antimetabolite

Questions 452–456

For each sign or symptom of disease listed below, select the disease with which it is most likely to be associated.

(A) Ventricular septal defect
(B) Aortic stenosis
(C) Tetralogy of Fallot
(D) Patent ductus arteriosus
(E) Coarctation of the aorta

452. Rib notching on x-ray and congenital berry aneurysm of the circle of Willis

453. Boot-shaped heart and a right-to-left shunt

454. Differential cyanosis if the shunt is reversed

455. Commonest cause of cyanotic congenital heart disease

456. May present with collapsing pulse and a "machinery" murmur in the second left intercostal space

Questions 457–461

For each treatment listed below, select the type of arthritis for which it would be most useful.

(A) Acute gouty arthritis
(B) Acute rheumatoid arthritis
(C) Lyme arthritis
(D) Osteoarthritis
(E) None of the above

457. Ascorbic acid

458. Penicillin

459. Hydroxychloroquine

460. Gold injections

461. Colchicine

Questions 462–466

For each definition listed below, select the term that it best describes.

(A) Pedophilia
(B) Voyeurism
(C) Transvestism
(D) Transsexuality
(E) Incest

462. Gender identity with the opposite sex

463. Intermittent but regular dressing by men in women's clothes to become sexually aroused

464. Sexual gratification from looking at sexual organs or sexual acts

465. Sexual interest in young children by an adult who is at least 10 years older than the child

466. Sexual activity between members of the same family

Questions 467–473

For each of the drug effects listed below, select the antigout medication that is most likely to cause it.

(A) Allopurinol
(B) Probenecid
(C) Colchicine
(D) Aspirin
(E) None of the above

467. Inhibits interaction between granulocytes and urate crystals

468. Inhibits xanthine oxidase

469. May precipitate gout if given in small doses

470. Produces a maculopapular rash

471. Drug of choice for recurrent urate nephrolithiasis

472. Drug of choice for acute gout

473. Inhibits active reabsorption of filtered urate

Questions 474–478

For each characteristic or sequela, select the disease with which it is most likely to be associated.

(A) Sarcoidosis
(B) Bagassosis
(C) Silicosis
(D) Asbestosis
(E) Berylliosis

474. Tuberculosis is a complication

475. Mesothelioma is an untoward effect

476. Noncaseating granulomas and ocular lesions are characteristic

477. Acute chemical pneumonitis may result

478. Hypersensitivity pneumonitis may result

Questions 479–483

For each type of cancer listed below, select the chemotherapeutic agent that is most likely to be effective.

(A) Diethylstilbestrol
(B) Mitotane
(C) Doxorubicin, radiation, and surgery
(D) Methotrexate
(E) None of the above

479. Wilm's tumor

480. Prostate carcinoma with metastases to the spine

481. Carcinoma of adrenal gland

482. Choriocarcinoma

483. Mycosis fungoides

Questions 484–488

For each antihypertensive medication listed below, select the untoward side effect with which it is most likely to be associated.

(A) Metabolic acidosis as a result of carbonic anhydrase inhibition
(B) Hirsutism
(C) Severe postural hypotension and syncope
(D) Rebound hypertension if treatment stops abruptly
(E) Cyanide toxicity with excessive dosage

484. Nitroprusside

485. Clonidine

486. Prazosin

487. Minoxidil

488. Acetazolamide

Questions 489–492

For each disease or untoward effect, select the etiologic agent most likely to be responsible for it.

(A) *Plasmodium ovale*
(B) *Entamoeba histolytica*
(C) *Trypanosoma cruzi*
(D) *Toxoplasma gondii*
(E) None of the above

489. Blackwater fever

490. Stillbirths and abortions

491. Hepatic abscess

492. African sleeping sickness

Questions 493–497

For each characteristic listed below, select the type of aneurysm that is most closely associated with it.

(A) Syphilitic aneurysm
(B) Atherosclerotic aneurysm
(C) Mycotic aneurysm
(D) Berry aneurysm
(E) False aneurysm

493. Associated with bacterial infection from an infected embolus

494. Found most commonly in the aortic arch

495. Usually occurs in the internal carotid artery

496. Is a congenital defect

497. Is traumatic in origin

Questions 498–500

For each definition listed below, select the term that it best describes.

(A) Sensation
(B) Perception
(C) Illusion
(D) Delusion
(E) Hallucination

498. Perception of an imaginary or interoceptive event as an exteroceptive reality

499. Fixed, false beliefs

500. Misinterpretation or misperception of actual environmental events

Section C

Answers and Explanations

ANSWERS AND EXPLANATIONS

1. The answer is A. (*Physiology Chapter 6 II A 3 b*) Gastrin, a product of the antral enterocytes, stimulates parietal cell secretion of hydrochloric acid, promotes gastrointestinal motility, stimulates exocrine secretion of pancreatic enzymes, evokes insulin secretion, and exerts a weak action on pancreatic water and bicarbonate (HCO_3^-) secretion. Secretin, which is synthesized by the duodenal and jejunal amine *precursor uptake* and *decarboxylation* cells (i.e., the APUD cells, or the enterocytes of the gastrointestinal mucosa), stimulates production of gastric pepsin (pepsinogen), evokes secretion of the inorganic components of bile by the liver, promotes insulin secretion, and stimulates the exocrine pancreas to release copious volumes of fluid with a high concentration of HCO_3^-. Secretin also inhibits gastrointestinal motility, which includes the relaxation of the lower esophageal sphincter. Other hormones that reduce lower esophageal pressure are gastric inhibitory peptide, glucagon, and cholecystokinin.

2. The answer is D. [*Anatomy Chapter 16 II E 2 a (2) (b); III C 1 b; V E 3; VI D 3 c (2) (a)*] The epiploic foramen (of Winslow) connects the lesser sac (the omental bursa) with the rest of the coelomic cavity (greater sac). The inferior edge of the ventral mesentery forms the epiploic foramen.

3. The answer is A. (*Immunology Chapter 1 II D 2 d*) Interferons are hormone-like glycoproteins produced by cells infected by viruses. Thus, interferon acts on neighboring cells by activating cellular genes to produce antiviral proteins that interfere with the translation of messenger RNA. Interferon also enhances T-cell activity, activates macrophages, and potentiates the cytotoxic action of natural killer cells. Interferons are nonantibody factors that contribute to natural immunity.

4. The answer is D. (*Behavioral Science Chapter 7 VII A 2; Chapter 9 V A 2; Chapter 12 VI A 3*) The death of a child is no doubt one of the most devastating experiences for any parent, particularly a sudden, tragic death as from a motorcycle accident. The anger expressed toward the physician by the man described in the question is a normal part of a grief reaction, as is his somatization of this intense emotional experience. Somatization can help this father to avoid temporarily the pain caused by the death of his son. Common complaints of patients who "convert" an emotional experience into physical symptoms include paralysis or failure of sight or hearing, paresthesias, vertigo, chest pain, hyperventilation, and palpitations.

5. The answer is E. [*Biochemistry, 2nd ed, Chapter 24 I B 1 a; Chapter 26 II A 3 b; Histology and Embryology Chapter 14 V B 2 a, b; Physiology Chapter 6 III A 5 b, B 3 c (2)*] Cholecystokinin (pancreozymin) is released from the enterocytes of the duodenum and upper jejunum mainly in response to the presence of protein and fat in the chyme. Cholecystokinin causes pancreatic cells to release large quantities of digestive enzymes that break down the proteins, carbohydrates, and fats present in the chyme. It also increases intestinal motility, causes gallbladder contraction, and stimulates insulin secretion.

6–8. The answers are: 6-D, 7-D, 8-C. (*Anatomy Chapter 29 II C 2; Physiology Chapter 1 XIII D 2 d*) The clinical presentation of a fixed facial expression, a "pill-rolling" tremor that is maximal at rest, rigidity, and passive movement of the limbs is the classic picture of parkinsonism. Parkinsonism can often be confused with other conditions.

Boxers are prone to develop multiple petechial hemorrhages in the brain. If major damage is in the substantia nigra, parkinsonism may develop. A lesion in the occipital lobe may be associated with visual disturbances, and a lesion in the temporal lobe may result in an expressive (Broca's) or receptive (Wernicke's) aphasia.

Pseudobulbar palsy may mimic Parkinson's disease, but hyperactive facial reflexes, pathologic emotionality, and spasticity distinguish it from parkinsonism. Tuberous sclerosis (Bourneville's disease) is associated with epilepsy, probably due to malformation of the cortex and calcification, especially in the temporal lobe seen on skull x-ray. Sycosis barbae is an infection of the hair follicles of the beard: It is not a neurologic condition. Catatonic schizophrenia is not associated with any tremor or abnormal reflexes.

9. The answer is D. [*Physiology Chapter 2 V A 2 a–d, e (1), f*] The lowest aortic pressure is seen at the end of the isovolumic contraction period, which marks the beginning of ventricular ejection and aortic systole. The mitral valve is closed during this entire period and opens at the end of isovolumic relaxation. The second heart sound marks the beginning of the isovolumic relaxation phase and the end of ventricular ejection and of aortic systole. The second heart sound is associated with semilunar (aortic) valve closure (incisura). The T wave of the electrocardiogram is completed by the end of the isovolumic relaxation period. Due to the increase in ventricular mural tension during the isovolumic contraction period, there is compression of the coronary arteries and reduced coronary flow. The correlates of the cardiac cycle are depicted in the figure below.

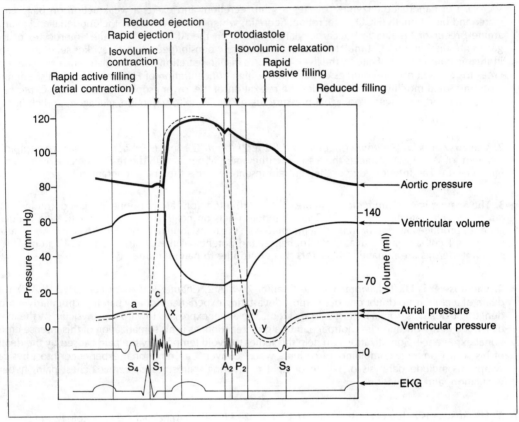

Reprinted with permission from Bullock J, et al: *Physiology*. Media, PA, Harwal, 1984, p 115.

10. The answer is D. (*Microbiology Chapter 17 III; Pediatrics Chapter 4 VIII B*) The patient in the photograph that accompanies the question has a dermatophyte infection known as ringworm (tinea corporis). It presents characteristically with circular lesions of varying size with slightly raised advancing borders and a light central area of healing, which may be erythematous. Dermatophytes affect only the nonviable keratinous structure of skin without penetrating deeper structures of the skin. Candidiasis is a dermatomycosis that can cause systemic disease. Pityriasis rosea is a self-limited nonfungal eruption of skin. Nummular eczema, an uncommon chronic dermatitis characterized by inflamed, discoid vesicular lesions, usually improves with corticosteroid treatment. Squamous cell carcinoma usually occurs in fair-skinned persons exposed to sunlight.

11. The answer is B. (*Anatomy Chapter 4 IV C 3 b; see also Appendix for references*) Lower motor neurons are fibers that innervate skeletal muscle, and when lesioned, there are deficits in motor function. These deficits include a flaccid paralysis, muscle atrophy, hyporeflexia, muscle fasciculations and fibrillations, and paresis. The paralysis may be complete (flaccid paralysis) or partial (paresis). Paresthesia, abnormal spontaneous sensations, such as numbness and prickling, results from lesions of the dorsal (sensory) roots.

12. The answer is D. [*Physiology Chapter 7 VII E 1 c (1) (a), (b)*] The substances found in seminal plasma can be correlated with the functional status of the testes because their synthesis depends on testosterone secretion. The seminal vesicles are the source of fructose, ascorbate, and prostaglandins, while the prostate synthesizes acid phosphatase, citrate, and fibrinolysin.

13. The answer is D. (*Anatomy Chapter 25 V A 2, B*) The anterior tibial artery enters the anterior compartment of the leg by passing above the superior margin of the interosseous membrane. It descends through the anterior compartment and enters the foot where it crosses the anterior aspect of the ankle and becomes the dorsalis pedis artery.

14. The answer is A. (*Physiology Chapter 2 VI A 1–3*) Poiseuille's law is summarized by the equation:

$$F = \frac{\Delta P \pi r^4}{8 \eta L},$$

where F = flow, ΔP = pressure difference, r = radius of vessel, η = viscosity, and L = length of vessel. From the equation, it is observed that flow is directly related to the difference in pressure and the fourth power of the radius, and flow is inversely related to the length of the tube and viscosity of the fluid. Further, resistance to flow is proportional to both the length of the tube and the viscosity of the fluid and is inversely proportional to the fourth power of the radius as:

$$R = \frac{8 \eta L}{\pi r^4}.$$

Reducing the length by a factor of 2 reduces the resistance by a factor of 2; reducing the radius by a factor of 2 *increases* the resistance by a factor of 16. Thus, the resistance is increased by a factor of 8 when considering the change of both variables together.

15. The answer is C. (*Immunology Chapter 9 III C; IV C*) Immune complex–mediated reactions are initiated by antigen–antibody (immune) complexes, which are either formed locally (i.e., at site of tissue injury) or are deposited from the circulation. These immune complex–mediated reactions are classically seen in Arthus reaction, serum sickness, hypersensitivity pneumonitis, poststreptococcal glomerulonephritis, and autoimmune disease. Erythroblastosis fetalis is a hemolytic anemia of the fetus or neonate due to a cytotoxic reaction initiated by maternal antibody reacting with cell-bound antigen (e.g., when a sensitized Rh-negative mother gives birth to an Rh-positive infant) acquired from an Rh-positive father. The sensitized mother has antibodies that enter the fetal circulation during pregnancy or parturition.

16. The answer is D. (*Histology and Embryology Chapter 8 II B 1–3*) The function of red blood cells is to transport oxygen and carbon dioxide. The delivery of these gases to and from the cells occurs across the capillaries—the exchange vessels of the cardiovascular system. Because of the small size of the capillaries, the red blood cells are deformed when squeezed through these small channels. The stress on the microvasculature contributes to the short life of the cells. After a life span of 120 days, red blood cells are removed from the circulation and destroyed by the reticuloendothelial system.

17. The answer is B. [*Physiology Chapter 1 IV A 1 b, c (1)–(3); Figures 1-15 and 1-18*] Individual myofibrils composed of myofilaments present a striated appearance of alternating light and dark bands. The wide dark bands, A bands, represent the region of thick parallel myosin filaments, and the white bands, I bands, represent the region of thin parallel actin filaments. The I band is bisected by a thin dark zone, the Z line. A narrow light region, the H zone, bisects the A band. The distance between two Z lines is a sarcomere. During contraction, opposing actin filaments slide toward each other over the myosin filaments, shortening the sarcomere and causing a narrowing of the I band.

18. The answer is A. [*Anatomy Chapter 19 III A 4 a, B 2 a (2); Chapter 28 IV A 2 b (1); Chapter 29 VI B 1 b*] The brain and spinal cord are suspended in a pool of cerebrospinal fluid (CSF) confined to the subarachnoid space between the arachnoid and pial (pia mater) meningeal layers. The CSF, a clear and colorless liquid, is actively secreted by the choroid plexus into the ventricular system at several points, but it is not a simple ultrafiltrate of plasma from which it is formed. CSF is being constantly formed (i.e., about 500 ml per day) and removed to maintain the constant volume of about 150 ml in the adult. Small elevations of the arachnoid (arachnoid villi) function as one-way valves, allowing CSF to be reabsorbed into the venous blood. The chemical composition of CSF is similar to plasma with the principal difference that plasma contains about 300 times as much protein as the CSF, which has a protein concentration of 20 mg/dl.

19. The answer is C. (*Pathology Chapter 5 II D 1 b; see also Appendix for references*) Syphilitic aortitis is almost always confined to the ascending and transverse parts of the thoracic aorta. The basic lesion is an endarteritis obliterans of the vasa vasorum supplying the aorta, which results in the ischemic destruction of the media with fibrous replacement, producing sacular and dissecting aneurysms of the ascending thoracic aorta, secondary aortic valve incompetence, and ischemic heart disease. This is a manifestation of tertiary syphilis. Syphilitic aortitis can cause angina pectoris, but it is indistinguishable from coronary artery disease due to atherosclerosis; however, syphilis is suspected when other manifestations of the disease are present.

20. The answer is C. [*Physiology Chapter 7 II C 2 a, b; IV B 2 a–c; V D 1 c (1) (a), (b)*] Somatomedin is a peptide but not a neuropeptide since it is synthesized mainly in the liver. Antidiuretic hormone, thyrotropin-releasing hormone, and oxytocin are secretory products of neurosecretory neurons. Endorphin has a wide distribution in the neurons of the central nervous system and the pituitary gland. It has also been found in the pancreas, placenta, semen, and in the male reproductive tract.

21. The answer is A. (*See Appendix for references*) Calcitriol (1,25-dihydroxycholecalciferol), the most active metabolite of vitamin D_3, contains 27 carbon atoms and is produced in the kidney from calcidiol (25-hydroxycholecalciferol). It is called a secosteroid because one of the four rings, the B-ring, is opened. It can function as parathyroid hormone in that it causes bone resorption (dissolution), which, in turn, increases the plasma concentration of ionized calcium in order to achieve normocalcemia. Therefore, this agent is used in the treatment of hypoparathyroidism.

22. The answer is B. (*Microbiology Chapter 21 I B; Pathology Chapter 13 IV A 2*) The lesion on the penis in the photograph accompanying the question is a simple wart—that is, condyloma acuminatum—a papovavirus infection. This viral infection is very common in sexually active men and women, but these lesions may also arise without sexual contact. Papovavirus is a DNA virus that is potentially oncogenic. The incubation period is 1 to 6 months. Attempts to propagate condyloma acuminatum in culture have been unsuccessful; the wart tissue is the only source of mature virus particles.

23. The answer is E. (*Physiology Chapter 1 XIII A, E, F 1 a, b*) Neurons originating in the cerebral motor cortex, the cerebellum, or the various brain stem nuclei that send axons into the brain stem and spinal cord to activate cranial and spinal motor neurons are termed upper motor neurons. Since the vestibulospinal tracts originate in the vestibular nuclei of the brain stem, they conform to the definition of upper motor neuron; thus, upper motor neurons belong to the somatic nervous system. The upper motor neurons form descending tracts in the brain stem and spinal cord. They are named according to their site of origin and the region of distribution. Cranial and spinal motor neurons are either somatic (i.e., they innervate skeletal muscle derived from mesodermal somites) or visceral (i.e., they innervate cardiac muscle, smooth muscle, or glands). The cranial and spinal motor neurons (somatic) that innervate skeletal muscles are the lower motor neurons, which are part of the peripheral nervous system.

The splanchnic nerve is an autonomic (sympathetic) motor nerve that innervates autonomic neuroeffectors. The supraopticohypophyseal (hypothalamoneurohypophyseal) tract is an unmyelinated tract consisting of magnocellular neurosecretory neurons that do not innervate any neuroeffector cells, but end on or near blood vessels. The sciatic nerve has both somatic motor and sensory nerves and, therefore, in part, contains *lower* motor neurons. The vagal efferents to the heart are autonomic motor fibers and, like the splanchnic nerve, are not lower motor neurons.

24. The answer is C. [*Biochemistry, 2nd ed, Chapter 17 II F 2 a; Physiology Chapter 7 VI H 1 a (1), b (2)*] Glucose-6-phosphatase is a gluconeogenic enzyme occurring in liver and kidney. Thus, muscle cannot synthesize glucose, and glycogenolysis in exercising muscle leads to an elevation of blood lactate. Indirectly, muscle contributes significantly to the level of blood glucose by providing the liver with an important gluconeogenic substance, lactate.

Muscle and liver contain glycogen phosphorylase, which is necessary for the depolymerization of glucose to form glucose-1-phosphate. These two tissues also contain phosphoglucomutase and phosphoglucoisomerase, which convert glucose-1-phosphate to glucose-6-phosphate and glucose-6-phosphate to fructose-6-phosphate, respectively.

Muscle, unlike liver, also lacks the glucokinase enzyme, which phosphorylates glucose to form glucose-6-phosphate. The phosphorylation of glucose in muscle is catalyzed by hexokinase, an enzyme with broad specificity and distribution.

25. The answer is C. (*Pathology Chapter 16 II I 7 a, b; Physiology Chapter 1 XIII D 2 d*) Parkinson's disease, a degenerative disorder that is often found in boxers, presents with tremors, rigidity, and hypokinesia. Mental processes are normal, but speech is slow and measured. The lesion responsible for this condition is caused by multiple petechial hemorrhages in the substantia nigra.

26. The answer is B. [*Physiology Chapter 7 IX E 3 a–c, F 1 a–c, 2 b (1), (2)*] The phases of the menstrual cycle are named in terms of ovulation, the pituitary, the ovary, and the endometrium. With respect to the midcycle surge in luteinizing hormone (LH), there are the preovulatory and postovulatory phases. When these phases are described with reference to the pituitary, they are called follicular (preovulatory) and luteal (postovulatory) because of the dominant secretion of follicle-stimulating hormone (FSH) and LH, respectively. In terms of the ovary, these same phases are called estrogenic (preovulatory) and progestational (postovulatory) because of the follicular secretion of estradiol and the corpus luteal secretion of progesterone, respectively. Lastly, when those phases are described with respect to the endometrium, they are termed proliferative (preovulatory) and secretory (postovulatory) to describe the regeneration of the stratum functionale and the secretory activity of the endometrial glands, respectively. In short, the four phases of the menstrual cycle are menses, preovulation, ovulation, and postovulation.

27. The answer is A. (*Microbiology Chapter 25 II B; see also Appendix for references*) Trichinosis is caused by the nematode *Trichinella spiralis*. Adult worms live in the intestines of humans, pigs, bears, rats, and most carnivores, including marine animals. Fowl, however, are resistant to infection. Larvae that are liberated by females enter striated muscle where they are encysted and live for years. In the natural life cycle, these larvae develop into a new generation of adults when parasitized muscle is ingested by a new host. Pigs generally become infested when they feed on uncooked food scraps or less often, by eating infected rats. Presenting signs of clinical disease include diarrhea, abdominal pain, malaise, periorbital edema, muscle weakness, and eosinophilia. Convulsions may result if the patient has cysticercosis, which is due to the pork tapeworm.

28. The answer is E. (*Physiology Chapter 2 V C 6 a*) The cardiac output, equal to the product of stroke volume and heart rate, can be determined by the Fick principle, which is used to measure blood flow through an organ. In this case, the Fick principle is used to calculate pulmonary blood flow. It is necessary to measure timed oxygen consumption and simultaneously the oxygen concentration in mixed venous blood (from the pulmonary artery) and in arterial blood. The cardiac output (pulmonary blood flow) is calculated as the quotient of the oxygen consumption (ml/min) and the arterial–mixed venous oxygen difference (ml/dl or ml/L). In this subject, the calculation is:

$$\text{Cardiac output} = \frac{300 \text{ ml/min}}{18 \text{ ml/dl} - 13 \text{ ml/dl}} = 60 \text{ dl/min} = 6 \text{ L/min}$$

$$\text{Stroke volume} = \frac{\text{Cardiac output}}{\text{Heart rate}} = \frac{6000 \text{ ml/min}}{75/\text{min}} = 80 \text{ ml}$$

Hematocrit is a distractor; it is not necessary for the calculation of stroke volume. Volumes percent is another expression for ml/dl.

29. The answer is E. [*Pharmacology, 2nd ed, Chapter 2 III B 1 a–d; Psychiatry Chapter 3 IV F 2 o (3)*] Propranolol, a β-adrenergic blocking agent, inhibits adrenergic mediators at their receptor sites in the heart and thus reduces heart rate and cardiac output. Propranolol is not a cardioselective β-adrenergic blocking agent and may block β_2 receptors of the bronchi; thus, it should not be given to patients with bronchial asthma. It also inhibits renin secretion. Other contraindications to propranolol include severe bradycardia, left ventricular failure, Raynaud's disease, and unstable diabetes prone to bouts of hypoglycemia. Although propranolol can cause excitement and confusion, it (and other β blockers) is often very effective in alleviating the palpitations, diarrhea, and tremor that accompany anxiety and apprehension. At moderate doses, it may produce lethargy and drowsiness. At high doses, other central nervous system complaints can occur, such as severe depression, psychosis with visual hallucinations, nightmares, and insomnia.

30. The answer is C. (*Biochemistry, 2nd ed, Chapter 11 IV D 1*) The Michaelis constant (K_m) is equivalent to the substrate concentration that yields half-maximal velocity. Since the maximal velocity, V_{max}, of this enzyme-catalyzed reaction is 120 nmol $\times$ L^{-1} $\times$ min^{-1}, the one-half maximal velocity, $V_{max}/2$, is 60 nmol $\times$ L^{-1} $\times$ min^{-1}. This corresponds to a substrate concentration ([S]) of 1.0×10^{-5} mol/L.

31. The answer is E. (*Biochemistry, 2nd ed, Chapter 11 IV C 3 e*) The rate of an enzyme-catalyzed reaction increases with substrate concentration until a maximal velocity (V_{max}) is attained, which in this problem is 120×10^{-9} mol $\times$ L^{-1} $\times$ min^{-1}. When there is a plateau of the reaction rate at high substrate concentrations, there is saturation of all the available binding sites on the enzyme. The best way to obtain V_{max} and K_m is to plot the data on graph paper. However, in this situation, we see that reaction rate (v) becomes relatively insensitive to changes in [S] above 2.0×10^{-3}M; that is, in the region of [S] = 2×10^{-3} to 1.0×10^{-2}M, velocity must be very close to V_{max}. It should also be noted that 1 nmol/L is equivalent to 10^{-9}M.

32. The answer is D. (*Biochemistry, 2nd ed, Chapter 11 IV C 3 e*) This problem can be solved simply by using the familiar Henri-Michaelis-Menten equation:

$$\frac{v}{V_{max}} = \frac{[S]}{K_m + [S]} \qquad \text{where velocity (v)} = \frac{V_{max}\,[S]}{K_m + [S]}.$$

Solving this equation with the data given yields the following:

$$v = \frac{V_{max}\,[S]}{K_m + [S]} = \frac{5000 \text{ mol} \times \text{min}^{-1} \times \text{mol}^{-1} \text{ enzyme } (3.0 \times 10^{-5} \text{ mol/L})}{3.0 \times 10^{-5} \text{ mol/L} + 3.0 \times 10^{-5} \text{ mol/L}}$$

$$= \frac{5000 \text{ mol} \times \text{min}^{-1} \times \text{mol}^{-1} \text{ enzyme } (3.0 \times 10^{-5} \text{ mol/L})}{6.0 \times 10^{-5} \text{ mol/L}}$$

$$= \frac{5000 \text{ mol} \times \text{min}^{-1} \times \text{mol}^{-1} \text{ enzyme}}{2}$$

$$= 2500 \text{ mol} \times \text{min}^{-1} \times \text{mol}^{-1} \text{ enzyme}.$$

33. The answer is B. (*Physiology Chapter 1 VI A, B*) Injury to the dorsal column is associated with (1) the inability to recognize limb position (i.e., loss of kinesthetic sense); (2) the inability to recognize familiar objects by touch alone (i.e., astereognosis); (3) loss of vibratory sense; (4) loss of two-point discrimination, and (5) inability to stand erect with feet together when the eyes are closed (Romberg's sign). Temperature information is conducted to higher brain centers via the contralateral spinothalamic tract.

34. The answer is D. (*Anatomy Chapter 10 Tables 10-1 and 10-2; IV D 2; VII C 3, D*) The "claw hand" deformity, the result of complete ulnar paralysis, is manifested by flexion at the interphalangeal joints, wasting of the small muscles of the hand, and hyperextension of the fingers at the metacarpophalangeal joints. The most common injury of the ulnar nerve occurs at the elbow; the ulnar palsy that results may be delayed for years after the injury. The ulnar nerve innervates the interosseous and lumbricalis muscles of the hand, causing flexion of the metacarpophalangeal joints and extension of the distal and proximal interphalangeal joints (DIP and PIP joints). When these muscles are paralyzed because of an ulnar lesion, the action of the long flexor and extensors become unopposed, resulting in hyperextension at the metacarpophalangeal joints and flexion of the DIP and PIP joints, resulting in classic "claw hand."

35. The answer is A. (*Physiology Chapter 1 XII C 4 a; Figure 1-55*) The motor (efferent) innervation of the intrafusal fibers of skeletal muscle is chiefly by gamma motor fibers. There is no gamma innervation of smooth muscle or tendons of skeletal muscle. Annulospiral endings and cutaneous touch receptors are innervated by sensory fibers. Muscle spindles contain two types of intrafusal fibers, both of which are multinucleated contractile cells. These two types are named nuclear bag fibers and nuclear chain fibers. Extrafusal fibers are the large contractile fibers of the muscle and are innervated by the large alpha motor neurons.

36. The answer is A. (*Biochemistry, 2nd ed, Chapter 28 I A 3, 4; Pharmacology, 2nd ed, Chapter 2 II A; Physiology Chapter 7 VI D*) Epinephrine is a catecholamine derived from the biosynthetic pathway beginning with phenylalanine or tyrosine as:

phenylalanine→tyrosine→dihydroxyphenylalanine (dopa)→dihydroxyphenylethylamine (dopamine)→ norepinephrine→epinephrine

It is a secondary amine synthesized mainly by the chromaffin cells of the adrenal medulla by the action of the epinephrine-forming enzyme (phenylethanolamine-N-methyltransferase) on norepinephrine, which is a primary amine. The methyl donor is S-adenosylmethionine. The human adult adrenal medulla secretes 85% epinephrine and 15% norepinephrine, making the adrenal medulla the major source of epinephrine.

37. The answer is A. (*Pathology Chapter 5 II C 3*) Buerger's disease (thromboangiitis obliterans) is an inflammatory disease of the arteries in which adjacent veins and nerves also become involved. Affected patients usually present with patchy thrombophlebitis of superficial veins. After the arterial lesion develops, patients complain of pain in the extremity, at first brought on by exercise and then during rest as well. Tissue ulceration and gangrene may result. Buerger's disease is very rare in women and in men who do not smoke. The etiology is unknown.

38. The answer is B. (*Physiology Chapter 3 III C 1, 2*) Since vital capacity is the maximal volume of gas that can be expired following a maximal inspiration (4.5 L), and the total lung capacity is given as 6.5 L, then the residual volume (RV) equals 2.0 L, that is, 6.5 L − 4.5 L. Since functional residual capacity (FRC) is comprised of expiratory reserve volume (ERV) and RV, then ERV = FRC − RV, or 3.0 L − 2.0 L = 1.0 L. It is important to note that in respiratory physiology a "capacity" denotes two or more "volumes." Pulmonary volumes and capacities are shown graphically below.

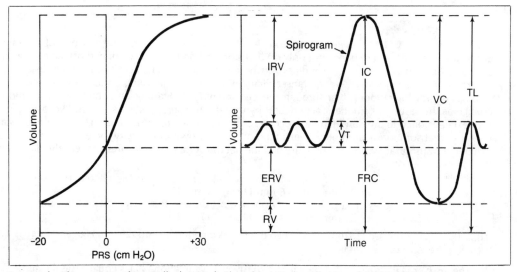

Reprinted with permission from Bullock J, et al: *Physiology*. Media, PA, Harwal, 1984, p 146.

39. The answer is E. [*Biochemistry, 2nd ed, Chapter 31 III E 5 a; Medicine Chapter 3 I B 3 a (1); Pathology Chapter 8 V F 7 a; Pharmacology, 2nd ed, Chapter 7 II C 1 b, 2 a; Physiology Chapter 6 II B 2 d (3)*] Vitamin B_{12} (cobalamin) deficiency may result from tapeworm infestation, purely vegetable diets, and intestinal blind loops with bacterial overgrowth. The most common cause, however, is a lack of intrinsic factor necessary for vitamin B_{12} absorption from the terminal ileum. Since intrinsic factor is a product of the gastric parietal cells and the ileum is the absorption site for this vitamin, both the stomach and ileum are necessary for vitamin B_{12} absorption. In the disease of familial multiple polyposis, the colon is studded with polyps. The appendix, and rarely, the ileum can also be involved.

40. The answer is D. [*Physiology Chapter 4 VI B 2 b (3)*] At plasma glucose concentrations below the renal threshold of 180 mg/dl (10 mM/L), glucose is completely reabsorbed and, therefore, has a clearance of zero. Urea is filtered at the glomerulus and variably reabsorbed so that its clearance is 40% to 70% of the true glomerular filtration rate. Inulin is completely cleared, and creatinine is filtered and secreted. Virtually all the potassium (K^+) is reabsorbed by the proximal tubule, whereas K^+ secretion is largely a function of the distal tubule.

41. The answer is B. (*Biochemistry, 2nd ed, Chapter 30 IV A 2, 6, C 1, 2; Histology and Embryology Chapter 16 I C 1 a; Pharmacology, 2nd ed, Chapter 10 IV B; Physiology Chapter 7 X A 2 b, C 1, 2, 6*) Insulin is a polypeptide hypoglycemic hormone, which is synthesized in the β cells of the pancreatic islet cells. It is composed of two chains connected by two disulfide bridges. The A chain is 21 amino acid residues in length, and the B chain is 30 amino acid residues in length for a total of 51 amino acid residues (MW of 6000). Insulin produces hypoglycemia by: (1) increasing glucose transport into muscle and fat cells, but it is not necessary for glucose transport into the liver, brain, lens, erythrocytes, and renal and intestinal epithelial cells; (2) activating glucokinase and glycogen synthetase, which phosphorylate glucose and cause glycogen deposition, respectively; and (3) promoting glucose utilization. Insulin is also a protein anabolic hormone because it increases amino acid uptake into muscle and enhances their incorporation into protein.

42. The answer is B. (*Physiology Chapter 5 II C 1, 2*) The classic description of the acid-base state, which is maintained by the lungs and the kidneys, is based on the Henderson-Hasselbalch equation, which is based on three variables (pH, P_{CO_2}, and $[HCO_3^-]$) and two constants (pK and S). The Henderson-Hasselbalch equation could functionally be written as:

$$pH = pK' + \log \frac{kidneys}{lungs}.$$

However, the equation is more usefully expressed as:

$$pH = pK' + \log \frac{[HCO_3^-]}{S \times P_{CO_2}}$$

or, using specific values for pK' and S, as:

$$pH = 6.1 + \log \frac{[HCO_3^-]}{0.03 \times P_{CO_2}}.$$

43. The answer is C. (*Physiology Chapter 2 I D 4 a, b; Chapter 4 V A 1 a, b*) The transport of substances across the capillary wall depends not only on diffusion and on the balance of hydrostatic and oncotic pressures but also on the structure and porosity of the wall and the characteristics of the substance being transported. The most important transcapillary exchange mechanism is diffusion, which can occur through intercellular "pores" or through the cell membrane. Starling described capillary fluid exchange as the result of osmotic (oncotic) and hydrostatic pressure gradients. When hydrostatic pressure exceeds oncotic pressure, filtration occurs, and when oncotic pressure is higher than hydrostatic pressure, reabsorption is promoted. Thus, fluid movement by transcapillary forces is the balance between net transmural hydrostatic pressure and the net transmural oncotic pressure. For the data given, the following equations apply.

Forces outward = capillary hydrostatic pressure + tissue oncotic pressure,
or 32 mm Hg + 6 mm Hg = 38 mm Hg.
Forces inward = capillary oncotic pressure + tissue hydrostatic pressure,
or 25 mm Hg + 4 mm Hg = 29 mm Hg.

Thus, the forces outward (38 mm Hg) exceed the forces directed inward (29 mm Hg), and there is a net filtration pressure of 9 mm Hg.

44. The answer is E. (*Physiology Chapter 3 IV B*) Alveolar ventilation ($\dot{V}_A$) is equal to tidal volume (TV) minus dead space volume (DS) times respiratory rate (RR), or

$$\dot{V}_A = (TV - DS) \times RR, \text{ but } \frac{DS}{TV} = 0.25.$$

Therefore,

$$DS = 0.8 \text{ L} \times 0.25 = 0.2 \text{ L}.$$

Substituting,

$$\dot{V}_A = (0.8 \text{ L} - 0.2 \text{ L}) \times 10$$
$$= 0.6 \text{ L/min} \times 10 = 6.0 \text{ L}.$$

45. The answer is C. (*Physiology Chapter 2 V C 4*) Afterload refers to the impedance to ventricular ejection and is equivalent to aortic pressure. The afterload at the instant of aortic valve opening (i.e., the beginning of ventricular systole) is equal to the aortic diastolic pressure (80 mm Hg).

46. The answer is E. (*Obstetrics and Gynecology Chapter 15 II E; Table 15-2*) All of the drugs listed in the question are teratogenic except penicillin. A fetal alcohol syndrome has been described that includes microencephaly, growth retardation, and short palpebral fissures. Tetracyclines cause staining of the deciduous and permanent teeth together with retardation of bone growth. In large amounts, vitamin A is teratogenic, causing central nervous system defects. There is an increased risk of congenital cardiac disease in infants exposed to lithium during early pregnancy.

47. The answer is E. (*Physiology Chapter 3 VII C 2*) Since there is an absolute decrease in the hemoglobin concentration in anemia, there would be a decrease in the amount of oxyhemoglobin and reduced hemoglobin concentration. The oxygen tension of arterial blood remains normal (100 mm Hg), while the oxygen content and oxygen capacity are subnormal. Since the erythrocytes generate large amounts of bicarbonate (HCO_3^-) by the action of carbonic anhydrase on carbonic acid, there is no increase in HCO_3^- formation with a decrease in the amount of hemoglobin in the blood.

48. The answer is B. (*Physiology Chapter 4 II C 3 c*) At the steady state, the osmolalities of intracellular fluid (ICF) and extracellular fluid (ECF) will be equal; however, the addition of 5 L of pure water to the

ECF will reduce the osmolality of that compartment. This will create an osmotic gradient in which water will move from a region of lower solute concentration (ECF) to a region of higher solute concentration (ICF). Also, it is essential to keep in mind that total body solute in this case remains constant. Therefore, we begin with 50 L of total body water at an osmolar concentration of 300 mOsm/L. This is equivalent to 50 L × 300 mOsm/L = 15,000 mOsm. With the increment of 5 L in the ECF (inulin space), there will follow a redistribution of water between the two major fluid compartments until the osmolar concentrations of both compartments are equal. It is not necessary to determine the new volume of each compartment. Therefore, the same 15,000 mOsm are distributed in a total of 55 L (50 L + 5 L), resulting in a steady state concentration of 15,000 mOsm ÷ 55 L, which is equal to 273 mOsm/L of total body water. The major body fluid compartments are presented in the diagram below.

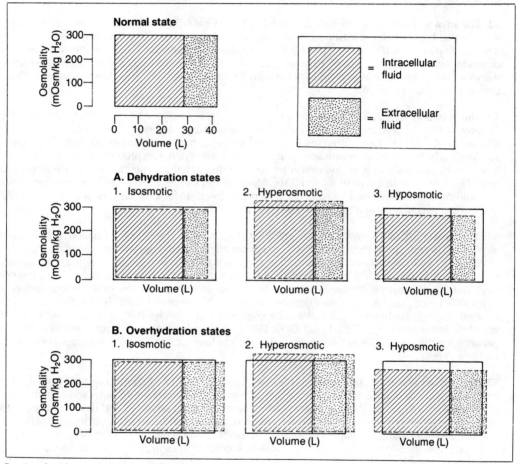

Reprinted with permission from Valtin H: *Renal Function: Mechanism Preserving Fluid and Solute Balance in Health*, 2nd ed. Boston, Little Brown, 1983, p 272.

49. The answer is B. (*Physiology Chapter 3 V B 2 a, C 2 c*) Pulmonary airway diameters increase at high lung volumes and with atropine, which blocks the bronchoconstrictor effect of the parasympathetic nervous system. When the terminal airways are considered in terms of *total* cross-sectional area, they are associated with a large total cross-sectional area and a decrease in airway resistance. On forced expiration, the airway diameters not only decrease (as they do during quiet breathing), but also the high velocity air flow leads to turbulent air flow and a further increase in airway resistance. Alveolar hypoxia is a potent constrictor of pulmonary blood vessels and results in increased pulmonary vascular resistance and pulmonary arterial pressure. Airway resistance falls dramatically as the alveoli are approached because the total cross-sectional area of the airways increases with each successive generation of branching.

50. The answer is C. [*Physiology Chapter 4 VI C 4 c (1)–(3); Chapter 5 VI D 1 a, E 3 b (1), (2)*] In acidotic states, ammonia serves as the major urinary buffer by combining with hydrogen ion (H^+) to form NH_4^+, which is excreted. It is important to emphasize that titratable acid does *not* include the H^+ that has combined with ammonia to form ammonium ion. Titratable acid is largely in the form of $H_2PO_4^-$, which is called acid phosphate or monobasic sodium phosphate. The two major urinary buffers are dibasic phosphate (HPO_4^{2-}) and ammonia (NH_3).

51. The answer is B (1, 3). [*Physiology Chapter 4 IX D 2 c (1) (a), e (2), (3) (a), (4) (a), (b)*] Sodium depletion stimulates the secretion of renin, which converts angiotensinogen to angiotensin I. This latter peptide is converted to angiotensin II, the aldosterone-stimulating hormone, by pulmonary angiotensin-converting enzyme. When angiotensin-converting enzyme is blocked, there is a decline in angiotensin II formation, a decline in aldosterone secretion, and a decline in sodium reabsorption. Concomitantly, there is an increase in renin secretion and in angiotensin I formation. The decline in the syntheses of angiotensin II and aldosterone would explain a decline in mean blood pressure.

52. The answer is B (1, 3). (*Pathology Chapter 10 III B 4*) Chronic active hepatitis is an inflammation of the liver that is present for at least 6 months. It is progressive and has a poor prognosis as most patients who develop cirrhosis die within 2 years from liver failure or hepatocellular carcinoma. It is seen more commonly in men over the age of 30 years. Most of the cases are of unknown etiology, although less than 50% of cases may be associated with hepatitis B virus infection (i.e., hepatitis associated with contaminated needles or blood).

53. The answer is A (1, 2, 3). [*Immunology Chapter 10 V H 2; Medicine Chapter 10 VI F 3 b; Pathology Chapter 11 III C 3 c; Pediatrics Chapter 7 V C 1 d; Pharmacology, 2nd ed, Chapter 3 III B 6 c, C 3 e (4); Chapter 5 IV E 2 d (3)*] Corticosteroids (e.g., prednisone) can improve a systemic lupus erythematosus–like syndrome. The anticonvulsants, primidone and phenytoin, can produce a rash that resembles lupus erythematosus and is an indication to stop the drug. Hydralazine can also cause a reversible lupus-like syndrome that is dose related. Procainamide also causes a reversible lupus erythematosus–like syndrome in approximately 30% of the patients on this drug for long periods, and as many as 70% of these patients may have a positive antinuclear antibody test.

54. The answer is E (all). (*Physiology Chapter 3 II C 1 d, 2 a, b, f*) The P_{50} is the PO_2 at which the hemoglobin is 50% saturated with oxygen. The hemoglobin affinity for oxygen is inversely related to the P_{50}. Thus, a shift of the oxyhemoglobin dissociation curve to the right brings about an increase in P_{50}. An increase in four factors will lead to an increase in P_{50}: PCO_2, hydrogen ion concentration [H^+], temperature, and 2,3-diphosphoglycerate (2,3-DPG). Therefore, an increase in any of these four factors enhances the unloading (i.e., increased delivery) of oxygen to the tissues. DPG is found in much higher concentrations in erythrocytes (15 mol/g of hemoglobin) and is synthesized by a shunt pathway in the glycolytic pathway from 1,3-DPG to 2,3-DPG. DPG, which stabilizes the deoxygenated form of hemoglobin, is synthesized at higher rates during alkalotic and hypoxic conditions. Hypercapnia denotes an increase in PCO_2.

55. The answer is A (1, 2, 3). (*Behavioral Science Chapter 2 IX D 4 b*) Opioids include both synthetic drugs and naturally occurring compounds, such as heroin, methadone, morphine, and codeine. In addition to being analgesics, these substances also cause euphoria, sedation, and decreased respiratory drive. A cross-dependence exists among opioids; thus, a patient addicted to heroin may be switched to methadone maintenance. A patient who is withdrawing from opioids is likely to present with rhinorrhea, lacrimation, piloerection, yawning, nausea, vomiting, sweating, diarrhea, abdominal cramps, and hypertension.

56. The answer is C (2, 4). [*Medicine Chapter 3 V D 2 a (2) (d); Pharmacology, 2nd ed, Chapter 7 III A 1 b, c (1), (2), 3, B 2*] Heparin, an antithrombin factor, does not block prothrombin *synthesis* in the liver as do the oral anticoagulants, but it does inhibit factors involved in the *conversion* of prothrombin to thrombin. Therefore, heparin interferes with the formation of fibrin. In contrast, the oral anticoagulants inhibit blood clotting mechanisms by interfering with the hepatic *synthesis* of the vitamin K–dependent clotting factors (i.e., factors II, VII, IX, and X). Heparin also inhibits the aggregation of platelets by thrombin. Heparin and the oral anticoagulants are inactive against thrombi once they have formed and, therefore, do not exhibit fibrinolytic activity. Heparin is found in mast cells and, therefore, is an intracellular glycosaminoglycan.

57. The answer is C (2, 4). (*Medicine Chapter 6 Part II I A 2; Pediatrics Chapter 15 IV B 1 a; Physiology Chapter 4 VII A 4, B 5, D*) The excretion of a hypertonic urine involves two basic processes: (1) the formation of a hypertonic medullary interstitium by the reabsorption of sodium chloride (NaCl) without water in the water-impermeable ascending limb of the loop of Henle and (2) the osmotic equilibration of the urine with the hypertonic interstitium as the urine enters the medullary collecting duct. Antidiuretic hormone promotes urinary concentration by increasing water permeability and urea permeability of the medullary collecting duct. It should be noted that the ascending limb of the loop of Henle is water impermeable and that water reabsorption is not an active process. Of the 1200 mOsm/kg solute concentration at the papillary tip during antidiuresis, half is composed of NaCl and half of urea.

58. The answer is B (1, 3). [*Behavioral Science Chapter 7 II A 2 b (4)*] Babinski's reflex is one of the simple reflexes possessed by the neonate. This extensor plantar response (i.e., hyperextension of the toes in response to stroking the sole of the foot) is normally present in infants up to 18 months of age and suggests an upper motor neuron lesion if present beyond 2 years of age. It does not, however, exclude an upper motor neuron lesion if it is absent in an adult.

59. The answer is E (all). [*Biochemistry, 2nd ed, Chapter 22 IV C 1; Pharmacology, 2nd ed, Chapter 8 IV B 1, C 1–3; Chapter 9 II B 1 b (1), 6 c; Surgery Chapter 1 V A 2 d*] The cyclooxygenase enzyme is inhibited by the nonsteroidal anti-inflammatory drugs (NSAIDs), such as aspirin (i.e., acetylsalicylic acid). Aspirin inhibits cyclooxygenase by the irreversible acetylation of this enzyme in platelets (i.e., thrombocytes), thereby preventing the formation of both prostaglandins and thromboxanes by these cells. The anti-inflammatory, analgesic, and antipyretic effects of NSAIDs are attributable to the inhibition of prostaglandins, especially PGE_2. The block in TXA_2 synthesis suppresses platelet aggregation, which, in turn, retards thrombus (i.e., clot) formation. Recent evidence suggests that low doses of aspirin (324 mg/day) are a useful prophylactic agent in preventing coronary embolization. This low dose may also allow the synthesis of prostacyclin (PGI_2) by endothelial cells. PGI_2 is a potent inhibitor of platelet aggregation. Since platelet aggregation plays a role in hemostasis, any reduction in the clumping of platelets results in the prolongation of bleeding time.

60. The answer is E (all). (*Physiology Chapter 1 VIII E 2 a*) Accommodation involves a triad of responses: (1) ocular convergence, (2) thickening of the lens, and (3) pupillary constriction (miosis). The thickening of the lens occurs through the contraction of the ciliary muscle, which decreases the tension on the lens. Convergence of the eyes is caused by the stimulation of somatic motor fibers of the oculomotor nerve that project to the medial rectus muscles that insert on the sclera. The oculomotor nerves also innervate the superior and inferior rectus muscles of the eyes. These muscles are the extrinsic ocular muscles, and the pupillary sphincter, radial muscle, and ciliary muscle are the intrinsic muscles (i.e., smooth muscle) of the eyes.

61. The answer is A (1, 2, 3). (*Anatomy Chapter 7 V B; Chapter 10 VII B*) The median nerve supplies all the pronation muscles of the forearm except the flexor carpi ulnaris and the ulnar half of the flexor digitorum profundus. The median nerve innervates the pronator teres, flexor carpi radialis, palmaris longus, flexor digitorum superficialis, radial half of the flexor digitorum profundus, flexor pollicis longus, and pronator quadratus muscle. Median nerve paralysis results in loss of pronation, weakness of abduction of the thumb, loss of light touch over the palmar aspect of the index finger, and thenar atrophy. Ulnar nerve paralysis causes hypothenar eminence wasting.

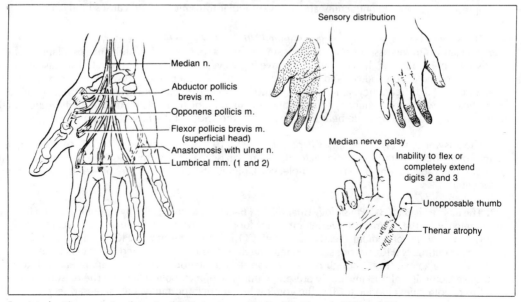

Reprinted with permission from April EW: *Anatomy*. Media, PA, Harwal, 1984, p 108.

62. The answer is B (1, 3). (*Physiology Chapter 7 VI E 1 a, b*) The secretion of norepinephrine (15%) and epinephrine (85%) from the adrenal medulla requires an intact neural input via the splanchnic nerves, which emanate from the intermediolateral gray column of the lower thoracic segments of the spinal cord. The adrenal medulla is the only autonomic effector that is innervated by preganglionic neurons, which, like all preganglionic neurons, are cholinergic in that they release acetylcholine. Acetylcholine depolarizes the chromaffin cells, which precedes the secretion of catecholamines. Interruption of the nerve supply to the adrenal medulla does not block the synthesis of adrenomedullary hormones, which depends on the secretion of cortisol from the adrenal cortex.

63. The answer is E (all). [*Biochemistry, 2nd ed, Chapter 17 I A 1, 2; Physiology Chapter 7 V D 1 c (4); VI H 3; VII F 1 a, b, d, f, 2 a (1), 3 a; X E 1 b, 2 b (1), 3 b*] The substrates for gluconeogenesis are noncarbohydrate precursors, which include all the intermediates of glycolysis and the citric acid cycle. These precursors are: lactate from erythrocytes and exercising skeletal muscle; glycerol from triacylglycerols in adipose tissue; and α-keto acids, such as pyruvate, oxaloacetate, and α-ketoglutarate from glycogenic (glucogenic) amino acids. Gluconeogenesis occurs primarily in the liver; that is, 90% of the glucose is made here. During prolonged starvation and metabolic acidosis, however, the kidney may contribute up to 50% of the glucose formed.

64. The answer is A (1, 2, 3). [*Medicine Chapter 1 I F 2 a, 3 g; II A 5 b (4) (d); Pharmacology, 2nd ed, Chapter 5 I A 8 c–e; Psychiatry Chapter 3 IV F 2 o (1); Surgery Chapter 3 V C 2 a–c*] Because of the inhibition of the sodium ion (Na^+), potassium ion (K^+)–adenosine triphosphatase pump by digitalis, there is a loss of intracellular K^+ and an accumulation of intracellular Na^+, which reduces the exchange of Na^+ for calcium ion (Ca^{2+}) and elevates intracellular Ca^{2+}. Digitalis delays conduction, an effect observed mostly in the atrioventricular node and manifested as an increase in the PR interval and a decrease in the rate of rise (slope) of phase 0 of the cardiac action potential. On the other hand, digitalis increases cardiac automaticity as seen by the increase in the slope of phase 4 (diastolic depolarization). There is also a decrease in the duration of the action potential plateau phase (phase 2), which reflects a shortened refractory period. This decrease in the rate of conduction and the shorter refractory period predispose the heart to reentrant arrhythmias, such as atrial or ventricular extrasystoles or ventricular fibrillation. In the atria and ventricles, digitalis shortens electrical mechanical systole, resulting in reductions of both action potential duration and QT interval. In summary, digitalis has the following effects on the cardiac action potential and the electrocardiogram: It increases the duration of both phase 0 and the PR interval; it decreases the magnitude and duration of the action potential; it decreases the transmembrane potential; and it decreases the duration of both phase 4 and the QT interval; extracardiac manifestations of digitalis toxicity include anorexia, nausea, and vomiting. Confusion and disorientation may be observed, especially in the elderly. Cardiac glycosides also have a vasoconstrictor effect on vascular smooth muscle, suggesting that myocardial ischemia can be a contributing factor to digitalis toxicity. Clinically, tachyarrhythmias associated with digitalis excess have been suppressed with propranolol. However, propranolol is not the agent of choice for digitalis toxicity because it depresses myocardial contractility and atrioventricular transmission and causes bradycardia.

65. The answer is C (2, 4). (*Physiology Chapter 1 VII B 3, C 2 a, b*) Oscillations in the air are converted into oscillations in the ossicles (i.e., malleus, incus, and stapes) and ultimately into oscillations of the fluids (i.e., perilymph) in the cochlea. The traveling waves are then transmitted to the basilar membrane near the *oval* window and then move along this membrane toward its apex near the helicotrema. High frequency sounds (e.g., 10,000 Hz) cause maximal oscillation of the membrane near the base while low frequency sounds cause the membrane to oscillate throughout its entire length but with the greatest amplitude near the apex where the width of the basilar membrane is widest.

66. The answer is D (4). (*Anatomy Chapter 17 VI D 5 d*) Cholecystokinin, which is secreted by the glands of the duodenal mucosa, stimulates the secretion of enzymes by the exocrine pancreas and gallbladder contraction. The release of cholecystokinin is stimulated by the presence of fat in the duodenum.

67. The answer is B (1, 3). (*Physiology Chapter 5 IX B 4; X E*) Normally, the hydrochloric acid (HCl) that is secreted into the stomach traverses into the duodenum where it stimulates the secretion of an equivalent amount of sodium bicarbonate ($NaHCO_3$). When the gastric HCl is eliminated from the body by vomiting, $NaHCO_3$ is not secreted into the duodenum but is retained in the plasma, producing a metabolic alkalosis. Even though potassium ion (K^+) depletion (hypokalemia) appears not to be a causative factor, it is almost invariably present in this type of metabolic alkalosis. The reason is not only the loss of potassium chloride (KCl) in the vomitus but, more importantly, the increased secretion of K^+

into the renal tubules and, hence, its increased excretion. Chronic renal failure and ketoacidosis are disease states associated with metabolic acidosis.

68. The answer is B (1, 3). (*Immunology Chapter 12 VI A, B*) Immunologically privileged tissues are sections of major blood vessels, bone, cartilage, and tendons that are used for grafting because they are never rejected irrespective of where they are transplanted. Nonvascularized tissue (e.g., the cornea) can also be used as a graft because there is little danger of immune rejection. There are also privileged sites, such as the brain, which tolerate grafting without sensitization of the recipient.

69. The answer is A (1, 2, 3). (*Medicine Chapter 5 IV D 4 b; Microbiology Chapter 24 III B 2–4, 6; Pediatrics Chapter 8 X C*) *Giardia lamblia* is the most frequently identified intestinal parasite in the United States. Giardiasis, the infestation of the small intestine by *G. lamblia*, is most prevalent in areas with poor sanitation and hygiene and is transmitted by the fecal–oral route. All age groups are affected with a large proportion of cases occurring in children in day-care nurseries and in homosexual men. Susceptibility to giardiasis is related to strain, virulence, size of the inoculum (fewer than 100 cysts cause infection), immunologic status of the host, and presence of hydrochloric acid in the stomach (i.e., patients with achlorhydria are more prone to infection). Giardiasis is successfully treated with metronidazole, quinacrine, or furazolidone (a liquid preparation).

70. The answer is D (4). (*Physiology Chapter 1 VIII E 2 a, 3*) An increase in pupillary diameter (i.e., mydriasis) is the result of the contraction of the radial eye muscles (iris), which is an α-adrenergic receptor response. The contractions of the ciliary muscle and the pupillary sphincter are controlled by the parasympathetic nervous system and are, therefore, mediated by cholinergic (i.e., muscarinic) receptors. Lastly, ocular convergence is controlled via the oculomotor nerve, which has somatic motor components and innervates the medial rectus muscles of the eyeball. The oculomotor nerves also innervate the superior oblique and superior and inferior rectus muscles. Thus, these extrinsic ocular muscles have cholinergic (i.e., nicotinic) receptors. The pupillary sphincter, the radial eye muscle, and the ciliary muscle constitute the intrinsic eye muscles, which are composed of smooth muscle. The sympathetic nervous system adapts the eye for far vision, while the parasympathetic nervous system adapts the eye for near vision (i.e., accommodation). Muscarinic receptors are cholinergic receptors found on structures innervated by either postganglionic parasympathetic neurons or by postganglionic sympathetic cholinergic neurons (i.e., sweat glands and vascular smooth muscle in skeletal muscle). Nicotinic receptors are cholinergic receptors on skeletal muscle innervated by somatic motor neurons or postganglionic soma innervated by preganglionic neurons.

71. The answer is E (all). (*Pathology Chapter 8 III F 1 a, b; IV C 2*) The carcinoid syndrome is due to a serotonin-secreting tumor that most commonly occurs in the terminal ileum (small intestine). These tumors can also occur in the appendix or bronchus. Carcinoid tumors are usually asymptomatic, but when active, they produce the carcinoid syndrome, which entails episodic flushing, abdominal cramps, diarrhea, and asthma.

72. The answer is A (1, 2, 3). (*See Appendix for references*) Zinc deficiency leads to growth retardation, delayed wound healing, gonadal atrophy, and impairments in taste (hypogeusia), smell (hyposmia), and appetite. As insulin is synthesized, the pancreatic β cell granule contents become electron-dense microscopically because the removal of the connecting peptide (C-peptide) from the proinsulin molecule decreases the solubility of the insulin molecule. In the presence of zinc, which is concentrated in the storage granule, insulin begins to precipitate as microcrystals of zinc–insulin hexamers. Crystalline zinc insulin is the basic pharmaceutical preparation of greatest importance in therapy. Zinc is an important component of many enzymes, including carbonic anhydrase, glutamic dehydrogenase, alcohol dehydrogenase, carboxypeptidase A, and RNA and DNA polymerases. Zinc deficiency is not related to hyperphagia.

73. The answer is E (all). (*See Appendix for references*) Mafenide is an anti-infective (i.e., antibacterial) skin preparation used topically to prevent sepsis and reduce morbidity and mortality in burn patients. It causes severe pain and delayed epithelialization at the site of application. Allergic skin reactions and acid–base disturbances may be encountered. The drug and its primary systemic metabolite inhibit carbonic anhydrase, leading to the loss of urinary bicarbonate ion and hyperchloremic metabolic acidosis. Compensatory tachypnea and hyperventilation with respiratory acidosis are also potential problems.

74. The answer is A (1, 2, 3). (*Physiology Chapter 4 IV D 2 a; VI A 1 b, 3 a–d*) Endogenous creatinine clearance is a common method used to estimate glomerular filtration rate (GFR) and, therefore, renal function. In this case the 24-hr creatinine clearance is given as liters per day and is equal to the GFR. The filtered load (i.e., amount filtered) of creatinine is estimated by the product of GFR and plasma creatinine concentration, or

$$150 \text{ L/day} \times 10 \text{ mg/L} = 1500 \text{ mg/day}.$$

Since the amount excreted (1700 mg/day) is greater than the amount filtered (1500 mg/day), the kidney must filter and secrete creatinine. The amount of creatinine secreted is the difference between the amount excreted and the filtered load, or 200 mg/day.

75. The answer is A (1, 2, 3). *[Anatomy Chapter 4 IV C 3 a; Chapter 29 II A 3 e (1)]* The cell bodies of the upper motor neurons lie in the gray matter of various nuclei in the brain stem and in the motor areas of the cortex. Fibers from these cell bodies pass through the cerebrum and brain stem and cross the midline in the lower half of the medulla and white matter of the spinal cord to contact the lower motor neurons (in the anterior horn of the spinal cord). Upper motor neuron lesions usually result in contralateral loss of abdominal and cremasteric reflexes and spasticity. Muscle wasting is not seen in upper motor neuron disease *except* long-standing hemiplegia where muscle wasting develops due to tissue atrophy. The lower motor neuron is intact; thus, galvanic and faradic stimulation produce normal reactions. Fasciculations, which are visible movements of muscle bundles, are a sign of *lower* motor neuron disease.

76. The answer is A (1, 2, 3). *[Medicine Chapter 10 II A 4 b (5) (a); Pharmacology, 2nd ed, Chapter 9 XI D 1 a]* Colchicine can be administered orally and intravenously only. However, it can cause gastrointestinal toxicity and should not be given orally if the patient has bowel inflammation. A major untoward effect is diarrhea. Colchicine can cause necrosis of the extravascular tissue if it leaks out of the veins. It also causes bone marrow depression if high doses are administered.

77. The answer is B (1, 3). *(Pharmacology, 2nd ed, Chapter 9 III F 3 b, c)* Acetaminophen poisoning (i.e., a single dose of more than 10 g in an adult or more than 3 g in a child) that persists beyond 24 hr causes a potentially fatal hepatic necrosis primarily in the centrilobular region, which may cause the prolongation of prothrombin time. Clinical symptoms, such as nausea and vomiting, occur during the first 24 hr after a toxic ingestion, while signs of hepatocellular damage (e.g., enzyme abnormalities) may not occur for 2 to 6 days. In turn, hepatotoxic effects may lead to encephalopathy, hypoglycemia, hemorrhage, cerebral edema, and death. Acetaminophen has little effect on respiration and, therefore, does not provoke hyperventilation as does aspirin. In contrast to the salicylate analgesics, therapeutic doses of aniline derivative analgesics (i.e., acetaminophen) do not cause gastric irritation or bleeding, do not possess anti-inflammatory activity, and cannot be used in the treatment of rheumatic fever or arthritis.

78. The answer is A (1, 2, 3). *(Immunology Chapter 1 II C 5, D 2)* Opsonins found in serum enhance phagocytosis; C3b, fibronectin, tuftsin, and antibody enhance the interaction between the engulfed particle and the phagocytic cell. Other opsonins include factors C5a, C5b67, and leukotriene LTBy. Their mechanism of action is by stimulation of chemotaxis. Beta lysin is an antibacterial nonantibody protein released from platelets when they are ruptured (e.g., in clot formation) and acts mainly against gram-negative bacteria.

79. The answer is A (1, 2, 3). *[Pediatrics Chapter I VI E 3; Chapter 2 IX F 4 b; Pharmacology, 2nd ed, Chapter 14 III B 3 d (1)–(8); Preventive Medicine and Public Health Chapter 12 IV A 4 c; Psychiatry Chapter 3 IV G 3 a]* Besides paint chips, the most common sources of lead include lead toys, storage batteries, ceramic dishes, and, in substandard housing, water pipes. Ninety percent of ingested lead is found in bones because lead is a "bone seeker." In addition to basophilic stippling of erythrocytes, lead produces a microcytic anemia as a result of impaired hemoglobin synthesis. Neural changes include demyelination and axonal degeneration in motor neurons, which impair neuromuscular function. Among the renal effects of lead toxicity are necrosis, atrophy, and renal interstitial fibrosis. Abdominal involvement includes pain, constipation, and colic. The appearance of a lead line on the gums is an indicative, but not invariable, sign of plumbism (lead poisoning).

80. The answer is A (1, 2, 3). *(Physiology Chapter 2 IX C 2 a–d; see also Appendix for references)* Trained athletes usually have a slower heart rate at rest and during a bout of exercise, in addition to having a larger stroke volume due to myocardial hypertrophy than nonathletes. This cardiac hypertrophy does not cause hypertension. Regular training also results in augmented cardiovascular efficiency, which is associated not only with enhanced oxygen delivery to the heart and peripheral tissues, but also with more efficient oxygen use by these tissues during exercise. Highly trained athletes have a lower resting heart rate of approximately 50 beats per minute, a greater stroke volume, a higher maximum oxygen consumption, a lower total peripheral resistance, increased capillary density in skeletal muscle, and greater extraction of oxygen from the blood (i.e., increased arterial–venous oxygen difference) by the skeletal muscle than nonathletes. The greater extraction of blood does not occur in the heart where increased oxygen demands must be met primarily by an increase in coronary blood flow.

81. The answer is A (1, 2, 3). [*Biochemistry, 2nd ed, Chapter 17 V B 2 b; Chapter 18 III F 1, 2 a; Chapter 30 II F 2 d; Pharmacology, 2nd ed, Chapter 2 II A 2 b (6), e; Physiology Chapter 7 VI G, H 1, 3*] Epinephrine produces hyperglycemia via the elevation of cyclic adenosine monophosphate (cAMP), which, in turn, activates phosphorylase activity in liver and muscle. This enzyme catalyzes glycogenolysis, which leads to glucose secretion by the liver. Muscle glycogenolysis leads to an increase in blood lactate (pyruvate), which is converted to glucose in the liver by gluconeogenesis. The hyperglycemic effect of epinephrine is augmented by its stimulation of glucagon secretion and its inhibition of insulin secretion. The latter effect is brought about via the α agonist activity of epinephrine on the β cells of the pancreas. Insulin *secretion* is stimulated via a β agonist activity.

82. The answer is A (1, 2, 3). [*Medicine Chapter 5 V F 2; Pathology Chapter 16 II J 4 f (3); Surgery Chapter 24 IV I 3 d, e*] Neurofibromatosis (von Recklinghausen's disease) is inherited as an autosomal dominant trait. It is characterized by multiple neurofibromas, café au lait spots on the skin, and Lisch nodules (hamartomas) of the nervous system and other organs as well. In approximately 8% of patients, malignant transformation of neurofibromas occurs. Polyposis coli is not a characteristic feature of neurofibromatosis. It may be associated with hereditary disorders, such as familial polyposis, Peutz-Jeghers syndrome, and juvenile polyposis, which may be associated with multiple polyps in the colon that carry a high risk of malignancy.

83. The answer is B (1, 3). (*Physiology Chapter 1 I C 1 a, b, 2 a, b*) The transport of glucose in the renal and intestinal epithelia occurs via a secondary active transport (cotransport) system, which is sodium ion (Na^+)–dependent. The Na^+ concentration gradient is the immediate source of energy for this process, but the transport of glucose is against a concentration gradient. The influx of Na^+ into the myocardial cells is accomplished by passive diffusion, while glucose transport into erythrocytes (and muscle and adipose tissue) occurs by facilitated diffusion. Both facilitated diffusion and cotransport processes are carrier-mediated transport processes; that is, they require a protein carrier. Notice that carrier-mediated transport systems can either be active or passive transport systems.

84. The answer is B (1, 3). [*Behavioral Science Chapter 7 II A 2 b (1); Pediatrics Chapter 16 Table 16-1*] Moro's reflex, or the startle reflex, involves the flexion of the extremities as a response to sudden stimulation. It is normally present in infants from 28-weeks gestation to 6 months of age. If Moro's reflex is present in infants older than 9 months of age, it suggests mental retardation and central nervous system abnormality. If this reflex is absent in neonates, it suggests severe central nervous system and brain stem disorders.

85. The answer is E (all). [*Pediatrics Chapter 16 V A 3 d (2), B 2; Table 16-4; Pharmacology, 2nd ed, Chapter 5 II C 2 a, 5 a, b, E 5, G 1 a, b, 4; Table 5-5; Psychiatry Chapter 3 IV F 2 o (2)*] The treatment of choice for ventricular tachycardia is direct current shock, but lidocaine, procainamide, or phenytoin are also efficacious. Lidocaine is particularly useful in controlling ventricular arrhythmias that occur during cardiac catheterization, myocardial infarction, and electrical cardioversion.

86. The answer is B (1, 3). [*Pharmacology, 2nd ed, Chapter 3 III B, C 3 a, d, e (5)*] The most common side effects associated with primidone therapy are related to central nervous system depression. Systemic lupus erythematosus, thrombocytopenia, leukopenia, rashes, megaloblastic anemia, osteomalacia, and personality changes (psychosis) have been reported. Gingival hyperplasia in children and hirsutism in young females are annoying side effects of phenytoin treatment.

87. The answer is D (4). (*Pathology Chapter 14 VIII E 1 a–c*) Sarcoma of the breast is an uncommon neoplasm, accounting for less than 1% of all breast cancers. Typically, breast sarcoma occurs in middle-aged women as a mass of soft consistency with prominent overlying vessels. These tumors are locally aggressive and metastasize through the blood vessels not the lymphatics. Early treatment by wide excision yields excellent results.

88. The answer is E (all). (*Histology and Embryology Chapter 10 V B 1–3*) The lymph node is surrounded by a capsule of dense collagenous connective tissue. It has a convex surface with several afferent lymphatic vessels entering it. It has one or two efferent lymphatics that drain the lymph node at the indented hilus, where blood also enters and leaves. See the figure below.

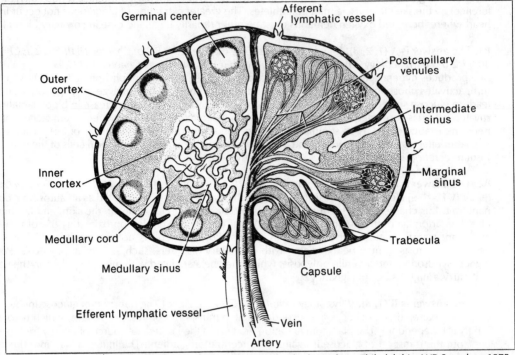

Reprinted with permission from Bloom W, Fawcett D: *A Textbook of Histology*. Philadelphia, WB Saunders, 1975, p 473.

89. The answer is A (1, 2, 3). [*Physiology Chapter 1 VI A 3 a (1), (2); Figure 1-26*] The important velocity-sensitive endings in glabrous skin are Meissner's corpuscles, which are a type of surface mechanoreceptor. These encapsulated nerve endings are found in the dermal papillae of hairless skin. Thus, they are classified as tactile end-organs and are located in the corium or subepidermal connective tissue of the palmar and plantar surfaces, forearms, lips, and glans penis. In humans, these receptors are most numerous in the skin over the fingertips. The receptors, which can be activated maximally by repeated stimuli at rates between 5 and 40 Hz, detect movement of a stimulus across the skin or of the skin across a surface. These receptors should not be confused with Meissner's plexus, a component of the enteric nervous system made up of ganglia and nerve fibers located between the submucosal layer and the inner circular smooth muscle layer of the gut. The enteric nervous system provides for coordinated movement of the gastrointestinal tract.

90. The answer is A (1, 2, 3). [*Biochemistry, 2nd ed, Chapter 22 I; II A; Immunology Chapter 9 II B 3 g; Medicine Chapter 7 II A 2 d (2) (d); Pharmacology, 2nd ed, Chapter 8 IV A, B*] Prostaglandins (PGs) are C-20 cyclic unsaturated fatty acids derived primarily from the essential fatty acid called arachidonic acid, a component of membrane phospholipids. Most mammalian cells, including endothelial and inflammatory cells, have the potential to produce PGs. They are found in exudates as a secondary response to the acute phase of inflammation. These ubiquitous substances are generally not stored in tissues.

91. The answer is A (1, 2, 3). [*Physiology Chapter 7 I D 1 c; V D 1 b (2) (a) (iii), (iv), d (7) (c); X A 4 c*] Somatostatin, a polypeptide hormone containing 14 amino acid residues, is synthesized in the parvicellular neurosecretory neurons of the hypothalamus, in the gastrointestinal tract, and in the δ cells of the endocrine pancreas. It inhibits the secretion of growth hormone, thyroid-stimulating hormone, glucagon, insulin, and gastrin. It also inhibits glucose absorption from the duodenum.

92. The answer is B (1, 3). (*Immunology Chapter 5 V B*) T lymphocytes are produced by a thymus-dependent system and provide "help" to the B lymphocytes to produce antibodies, but T lymphocytes do not themselves produce antibodies. Antigen recognition by T lymphocytes is specific but is not mediated by immunoglobulins. T lymphocytes populate the deep cortex of the lymph node and are not phagocytic as are the neutrophils and fixed macrophages that occur in the spleen (dendritic cells) and liver (Kupffer's cells). T lymphocytes, which comprise about two-thirds of the circulating lymphocytes, are small and medium-sized with a life span of up to 5 years. Activated T lymphocytes mediate *cellular* immunity either by a direct toxic effect through a reaction with the cell membrane–associated antigens or through the release of soluble factors called lymphokines. The larger B lymphocytes, which are derived from bone marrow and comprise about one-third of blood lymphocytes, are short-lived, having a life span of 5 to 7 days. They are responsible for the production of humoral antibodies, following their transformation into antibody-producing cells.

93. The answer is A (1, 2, 3). [*Pharmacology, 2nd ed, Chapter 5 I A 8 e; Psychiatry Chapter 3 IV F 2 o (1)*] Administration of toxic doses of digitalis results in large net losses of intracellular potassium ion (K^+), which, in turn, reduces the resting membrane potential of cardiac myocytes, resulting in the appearance of extrasystoles. Extracardiac manifestations of toxicity include gastrointestinal disturbances with anorexia, nausea, and vomiting as the most common. Diarrhea occurs rarely. Fatigue is the most common neurologic symptom of toxicity. Other symptoms include depression, drowsiness, weakness, restlessness, nightmares, headache, personality changes, vertigo, and confusion. Ocular disturbances include blurred vision, photophobia, xanthopsia, visions of flashing lights, scotomata, and amblyopia. Sydenham's chorea, which consists of simple chorea with irregular involuntary movements of the face and extremities, does not occur in digitalis toxicity.

94. The answer is E (all). [*Behavioral Science Chapter 7 II B 6 b (2)*] Aspects of psychological development between 18 months and 3 years include play, autonomy, self-awareness, and gender identity. Play provides pleasure and a means of reducing tension. Between 18 and 36 months, the child increasingly attempts to separate psychologically from the mother. As a means of achieving autonomy, the child manifests noncompliant behaviors, and resists parental authority. By 18 months, a relatively stable core gender identity (i.e., sense of being a boy or a girl) is established through experience and expectations. There is also an increasing sense of self as a separate individual within the confines of the family.

95. The answer is C (2, 4). (*Physiology Chapter 3 VII C 1; Chapter 5 VIII D 2; IX B 2*) The excessive elimination of CO_2 (hyperventilation) is the primary cause of respiratory alkalosis. Note that the concentration of hydrogen ion ($[H^+]$) and bicarbonate ion ($[HCO_3^-]$) change (decrease) in the same direction, a finding pathognomonic of respiratory alkalosis. The $[HCO_3^-]$ to ($S \times P_{CO_2}$) ratio is higher than normal [i.e., 19 mEq/L ÷ (0.03 × 20 mm Hg), or 19 ÷ 0.6 = 31.7]. Clearly, this patient has a reduction in CO_2 content. Compensation, if present, occurs in the alternate variable in the same direction. Thus, compensation for respiratory alkalosis would take place through the renal excretion of HCO_3^-. There is partial renal compensation in this patient. Since this patient has a P_{O_2} of 40 mm Hg, there is no hypemic hypoxia present because the P_{O_2} in hypemic hypoxia is normal. Hypoxic hypoxia is the only type of hypoxia associated with a decrease in the P_{O_2} of arterial blood.

96. The answer is B (1, 3). [*Medicine Chapter 7 III F 2 c; Pediatrics Chapter 7 IV A 3 b; Chapter 11 III F 1 c (3); Pharmacology, 2nd ed, Chapter 8 V A 1 e (2) (a), (b)*] Cromolyn is not a bronchodilator. It has no discernible effect on smooth muscle nor does it antagonize the effects of the chemical mediators responsible for an asthmatic attack. Thus, it has no sympathomimetic, antihistaminic, or corticosteroid-like actions. Instead, it prevents the antigenically induced tissue release of histamine and other spasmogens (e.g., leukotrienes), following immunologic (e.g., antigen–antibody) and nonimmunologic (e.g., exercise or hyperventilation) stimulation. It is effective when it is used prophylactically and should not be used to manage acute episodes of bronchospasm.

97. The answer is C (2, 4). (*Microbiology Chapter 25 I C; II B; see also Appendix for references*) Trichuriasis is caused by *Trichuris trichiura*, a common intestinal parasite (whipworm) in humans. The whipworm has characteristic barrel-shaped eggs, and, thus, the diagnosis is made by identifying the eggs in the stool. Most infections are asymptomatic, but the patient may develop dyspepsia, diarrhea, and rectal prolapse. Periorbital and facial edema, dyspepsia, muscle tenderness, eosinophilia, and a history of ingestion of undercooked pork (including boar) or bear meat are associated with trichinosis caused by *Trichinella spiralis*.

98. The answer is D (4). [*Physiology Chapter 7 IX E 1 b (3)*] The menopause is characterized, in part, by the elevation of plasma levels of the gonadotropic hormones, follicle-stimulating hormone (FSH) and luteinizing hormone (LH). Since there is a decline of ovarian function with menopause, the hypogonadism is due to primary ovarian failure. Thus, the inability of the ovaries to respond to FSH and LH is considered an end-organ insensitivity. The endometrium is still capable of responding to estrogens (e.g., estradiol) and progestins (e.g., progesterone); however, with ovarian failure, there is a marked decline in the synthesis and secretion of these steroids.

99. The answer is A (1, 2, 3). [*Pharmacology, 2nd ed, Chapter 2 II A 4 b (2), B 1 c, d, 2 c; Chapter 3 VII B 2 d (2), e, h; Psychiatry Chapter 1 VII B 2 a (1); Chapter 2 VIII A 3 b (4); Chapter 3 IV F 2 j (3); Chapter 5 VII C 3*] Monoamine oxidase inhibitors (MAO inhibitors) are used much less frequently than tricyclic and related antidepressants because of the dangers of dietary and drug interactions. MAO inhibitors cause an accumulation of sympathomimetic neurotransmitters, which can result in serious hypertensive crises. Sympathomimetics are present in some over-the-counter drugs, such as cough mixtures and decongestant nasal drops. Additionally, all patients should be warned against eating foods with high tyramine content, such as aged cheeses, sour cream, pickled herring, broad bean pods, yogurt, liver, yeast extracts, canned figs, raisins, as well as such beverages as wine, beer, sherry, and coffee. Other groups of drugs whose effects are augmented by the MAO inhibitors include central nervous system depressants (e.g., barbiturates), narcotics, anticholinergic agents, and hypotensive drugs. Large doses of isoproterenol (i.e., isoprenaline) can produce such excessive cardiac stimulation combined with a decrease in diastolic pressure that coronary insufficiency, arrhythmias, and ventricular fibrillation may result. Orthostatic hypotension is a common side effect of MAO inhibitors. Cardiac arrhythmias and heart block occasionally follow the use of tricyclic antidepressants, particularly amitriptyline. MAO inhibitors intensify the effects of tricyclic antidepressants.

Propranolol does not cause any adverse drug interactions, and, in fact, is often used to treat hypertensive crises that may occur in patients on MAO inhibitors.

100. The answer is A (1, 2, 3). (*Biochemistry, 2nd ed, Chapter 28 II E; Physiology Chapter 6 III E 7 c*) Ingested iron is reduced from the ferric (Fe^{3+}) state to the ferrous (Fe^{2+}) state in the stomach and upper intestine. Absorption is most efficient in the duodenum and upper small intestine. Ascorbic acid (vitamin C) facilitates iron absorption by reducing it to the ferrous state. Iron overload (hemosiderosis) produces gastrointestinal ulcerations, nausea, vomiting, abdominal pain, and diarrhea. Systemic effects of iron excess include acidosis, shock, drowsiness, coma, respiratory failure, and liver damage. Loss of iron from the body is about 0.5 to 1.0 mg per day in feces, urine, and sweat. An additional similar amount per day is lost by menstruating women during a normal menses.

101. The answer is A (1, 2, 3). (*Medicine Chapter 9 III A 6; Table 9-7; Pathology Chapter 11 VIII B*) Hypernephromas are renal cell carcinomas that are found in the proximal convoluted tubule; their etiology is unknown, although they have been produced experimentally using viral, chemical, and physical agents. Hypernephroma classically produces hematuria, pain, and flank mass; however, other symptoms include fever and vena caval obstruction, resulting in collateral circulation and leg edema. It also causes hypercalcemia, not hypocalcemia.

102. The answer is E (all). (*Physiology Chapter 2 V C 6; see also Appendix for references*) Cardiac output, the product of cardiac rate and stroke volume, is approximately 5 L/min in a normal adult. With maximal exercise, it increases to about 15–20 L/min in a normal adult. In a trained athlete, cardiac output may increase to 30 L/min during strenuous exercise.

103. The answer is A (1, 2, 3). [*Anatomy Chapter 30 I B 5 a (4) (b); Chapter 32 III A 7; Pediatrics Chapter 16 XI F 2*] Bell's palsy is probably a postinfectious neuropathy, usually due to inflammation of the nerve in the facial canal, resulting in paralysis of the muscles of expression on the same side as the lesion. This causes an ipsilateral expressionless drooping of the face. There is also ipsilateral paralysis of the orbicularis oculi, which causes an inability to close the eyelids completely, resulting in epiphora (i.e., impaired lacrimation) with conjunctival and corneal ulceration. Orbicularis oris paralysis results in drooling and difficulty in mastication. Chorda tympani involvement results in loss of taste in the anterior two-thirds of the tongue and reduced salivary secretion ipsilaterally. Hyperacusis results when the nerve to the stapedius muscle is also affected.

104. The answer is E (all). (*Pharmacology, 2nd ed, Chapter 5 II B 2, 3, 5, 7 a*) The major uses of quinidine are: (1) to maintain a normal sinus rhythm; (2) to prevent frequent premature ventricular contractions (PVCs) or paroxysmal ventricular tachycardia; and (3) to prevent arrhythmias associated with electrical countershock. Quinidine depresses myocardial contractility, which, together with its peripheral vasodilator effect, produces severe hypotension. Other manifestations of cardiac toxicity are atrioventricular block; prolonged PR, QRS, and QT intervals; and ventricular tachyarrhythmias. Quinidine has both direct and indirect (i.e., anticholinergic) effects on the heart. It depresses automaticity, particularly in ectopic sites; retards conduction velocity; and increases the effective refractory period of myocardial cells.

105. The answer is A (1, 2, 3). (*Histology and Embryology Chapter 17 IV B 5; V; Chapter 24 V A 1*) Melanin, the pigment that is responsible for skin, hair, and eye color, is found in melanocytes, which are normally found in the dermoepithelial interface, in the hair bulb, the uveal tract, retinal pigment epithelium, and the leptomeninges. The zona pellucida is found in the ovarian follicle and contains no melanin.

106. The answer is D (4). (*Physiology Chapter 3 VI A 2, B 1 b, C 2*) Both the blood flow, or perfusion, and the alveolar ventilation are lower at the apex of the lung than they are at the base. However, the decline in perfusion from the bottom of the lung to the top is steeper than the decline in ventilation. Because of this, the ventilation–perfusion ratio is relatively low at the base of the lung and much higher in the upper regions of the lung. This means that the base of the lung is relatively overperfused and the apex of the lung is relatively overventilated. When ventilation exceeds blood flow, alveolar P_{CO_2} decreases, and the alveolar P_{O_2} increases. The relationship between alveolar ventilation and pulmonary blood flow in the normal lung is summarized in the figure below.

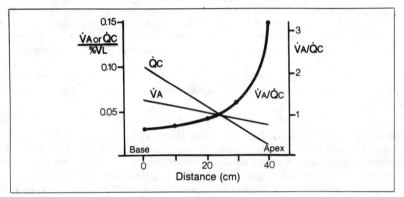

Adapted from West JB: *Ventilation/Blood Flow and Gas Exchange*. Oxford, Blackwell Scientific, 1970, p 33.

107. The answer is A (1, 2, 3). (*Pharmacology, 2nd ed, Chapter 2 IV F; Chapter 3 IV C; V A 3, D; Table 3-2; Physiology Chapter 1 XIII D 2 d; Psychiatry Chapter 1 VIII H 1 f; Table 1-3*) Antipsychotic drugs are also known as neuroleptics and, misleadingly, as tranquilizers. These drugs act by interfering with dopaminergic transmission in the limbic, nigrostriatal, and hypothalamic systems by blocking dopaminergic receptors, which give rise to extrapyramidal symptoms with chronic administration. Thus, the phenothiazines (e.g., trifluoperazine) and the butyrophenones (e.g., haloperidol) are antipsychotic agents while the antispasmotic agent, metoclopramide, is a cholinergic agonist. All three of these drugs can induce the extrapyramidal reactions of parkinsonism. Amantadine is an antiviral compound that is also useful in the treatment of Parkinson's disease because it evokes the release of dopamine in the substantia nigra and blocks its re-uptake.

108. The answer is B (1, 3). (*Biochemistry, 2nd ed, Chapter 28 II D 3 a–c; Pharmacology, 2nd ed, Chapter 12 II G 7; Physiology Chapter 6 III C 6*) Bilirubin is noncovalently bound to albumin and transported to the liver where it dissociates from the albumin and enters a hepatocyte. Within the endoplasmic reticulum of the hepatocyte, bilirubin is converted to a water-soluble glucuronide conjugate through the action of glucuronyl transferase. The mammalian placenta is capable of rapidly transporting bilirubin from the fetal to the maternal circulation and thus serves to rid the fetus of bilirubin. An untoward effect of the sulfonamides is kernicterus, which can occur in the newborn because of the displacement of bilirubin from plasma albumin. Kernicterus refers to the destructive deposition of bilirubin in the brain and nervous system and is more likely to occur in preterm than term infants.

109. The answer is A (1, 2, 3). (*Physiology Chapter 4 IV B 1; V C 3; VI A 3, B 3 c*) Measurement of renal function of the subject described in the question revealed the following data:

(1) Glomerular filtration rate (GFR) = $\dfrac{U_{in} \times \dot{V}}{P_{in}} = \dfrac{150\ mg/ml \times 1.1\ ml/min}{1.25\ mg/ml} = \dfrac{165\ ml/min}{1.25} = 132\ ml/min.$

(2) Filtered load of glucose = GFR × P_G = 132 ml/min × 0.8 mg/ml = 106 mg/min.

(3) Renal blood flow (RBF): Since the transport of inulin is 0, then:

$$GFR \times P_{in} = \text{Renal plasma flow (RPF)} (A_{in} - V_{in})$$

$$RPF = \frac{GFR \times P_{in}}{A_{in} - V_{in}} = \frac{132 \text{ ml/min} \times 1.25 \text{ mg/ml}}{1.25 - 1.00 \text{ mg/ml}} = 660 \text{ ml/min}.$$

(4) $RBF = \dfrac{RPF}{1 - Hct} = \dfrac{660 \text{ ml/min}}{0.55} = 1200 \text{ ml/min}.$

(5) Filtration fraction $= \dfrac{GFR}{RPF} = \dfrac{132 \text{ ml/min}}{660 \text{ ml/min}} = 0.2.$

110. The answer is E (all). [*Medicine Chapter 1 II A 4 b (1), 5 b (5); VII A 5 b; Chapter 2 VII G 2; Microbiology Chapter 8 II D 6; Pharmacology, 2nd ed, Chapter 7 III C 5 a, b; Surgery Chapter 13 V D 5; Chapter 14 II F 3*] Fibrinolysis requires the conversion of the inactive proenzyme plasminogen, which is present in clots and in plasma, to plasmin (i.e., fibrinolysin), a proteolytic enzyme not normally present in blood. Plasmin catalyzes the hydrolysis of fibrin, fibrinogen, and other blood clotting factors. The conversion of plasminogen to plasmin normally is initiated by tissue plasminogen factor, which is synthesized by the endothelium and released into the circulation. Streptokinase is a thrombolytic agent that brings about lysis of acute deep vein and pulmonary emboli and acute arterial thrombi. It has also been used for debriding surface infections, treatment of fibrinous exudates, and enhancement of wound healing in addition to lysis of intravascular clots. Streptokinase, unlike urokinase, can evoke allergic reactions and is contraindicated in streptococcal infections because it is produced by streptococci of groups A and C.

111. The answer is A (1, 2, 3). [*Histology and Embryology Chapter 23 III A 1; IV A 2; Physiology Chapter 4 IX D 2 a (1), (2)*] The juxtaglomerular cells, which are specialized myoepithelial (modified smooth muscle) cells located in the media of the afferent arterioles, synthesize, store, and secrete a proteolytic enzyme called renin. Bowman's capsule is a distended epithelial structure with a deep indentation that engulfs the vascular tufts of fenestrated capillaries called glomeruli. Bowman's capsules of the 10^6 nephrons found in each kidney are located in the renal cortex. Since each Bowman's capsule is occupied by a glomerulus, all of the afferent arterioles also are found in the renal cortex. Therefore, renin is selectively localized in the juxtaglomerular cells of the afferent arterioles within the renal cortex. The macula densa cells, which are specialized renal tubular cells located at the transition between the thick segment of the nephron and the distal convoluted tubule, do not secrete renin.

112. The answer is E (all). [*Pharmacology, 2nd ed, Chapter 5 IV G 2 f (2), (4), (7); Psychiatry Chapter 3 IV F 2 o (5)*] Methyldopa enters the brain where it is converted to α-methylnorepinephrine and is then released. The α-methylnorepinephrine activates the central nervous system α-adrenergic receptors whose function is to decrease sympathetic outflow, resulting in a hypotensive effect. Thus, it is classified as a centrally acting antihypertensive drug. Edema caused by salt and water retention can occur in the absence of a diuretic. Lactation (i.e., galactorrhea) can occur in both sexes, and impotence is observed in some men. Alterations in liver function may be accompanied by fever and malaise, which are indicative of hepatitis.

113. The answer is A (1, 2, 3). (*Biochemistry, 2nd ed, Chapter 17 V B 1, 2; Physiology Chapter 7 VI H 1, 3; X C 1 d*) Hypoglycemia evokes the secretion of epinephrine and glucagon. In turn, epinephrine stimulates glycogenolysis, especially in muscle, thereby providing lactate for hepatic gluconeogenesis. Similarly, glucagon stimulates hepatic gluconeogenesis. In contrast, these two hormones have opposite effects on insulin secretion in that epinephrine inhibits, while glucagon stimulates, insulin secretion. Insulin tends to decrease blood glucose concentrations by increasing glucose utilization, and promoting glycogen formation.

114. The answer is A (1, 2, 3). [*Physiology Chapter 1 II C 4; III C 2 b, c; V B 1; Chapter 2 II B 2, 3 c (5)*] The local current spreads only a very short distance through the axoplasm before flowing out through the membrane, *partially* depolarizing it, and producing an electrotonic potential. Electrotonic potentials are only observed when the intensity of the stimulus is *subthreshold* because once the excitatory threshold is reached, the electrotonic potential is obliterated by the formation of an action potential. Thus, electrotonic potentials are subthreshold, localized, nonpropagated, and proportional to the stimulus intensity. Since they are subthreshold, it is possible to summate electrotonic potentials.

115. The answer is A (1, 2, 3). (*Physiology Chapter 5 II C; IV A, B; VI; Table 5-7*) The Henderson-Hasselbalch equation (pH = 6.1 + log [HCO_3^-]/S × P_{CO_2}) is an expression of the three variables (pH, P_{CO_2}, and [HCO_3^-]) and two constants (pK and S) in the acid–base state. It basically can be interpreted as follows: The greater the concentration of dissolved carbon dioxide ([CO_2]), the lower the pH, and the greater the bicarbonate ion concentration ([HCO_3^-]), the higher the pH. The Henderson-Hasselbalch equation represents the bicarbonate buffer system, which is quantitatively the most important buffer of noncarbonic acid. Total CO_2 content is mainly the sum of [HCO_3^-] and dissolved CO_2.

116. The answer is C (2, 4). (*Pathology Chapter 14 VIII A 1, 3 b, 4*) Breast cancer is most common in the upper outer quadrant of the left breast. It has been hypothesized that the upper outer quadrant is more susceptible because it contains the greatest volume of mammary tissue. Carcinoma of the breast is commoner in women with a prior history of breast carcinoma—that is, the other breast has a high risk of developing breast carcinoma de novo, not just from lymphatic spread. Breast cancer is more common in women who have delayed childbearing (late first pregnancy); a familial history of breast cancer; a previous history of papillomatosis, uterine cancer, or epithelial hyperplasia; a history of chronic estrogen administration for more than 10 to 12 years; early menarche (under age 12); and a late menopause (beyond age 50). Eighty percent of breast cancers occur in women older than 40 years of age. Of these, 80% arise from the ductal epithelia and are, therefore, adenocarcinomas.

117. The answer is A (1, 2, 3). (*Pharmacology Chapter 3 VI A 5 e; see also Appendix for references*) Goiter with or without hypothyroidism is sometimes encountered in patients who are receiving lithium as a treatment for a psychiatric condition. Lithium, like iodide, decreases thyroid hormone synthesis. Other drugs that have been reported to produce goitrous hypothyroidism include para-aminosalicylic acid and phenylbutazone. Like the commonly used antithyroid agents, these drugs exert their effect by interfering with both the organ-binding of iodine and the later steps in thyroid hormone biosynthesis. This results in increased thyroid-stimulating hormone stimulation of thyroid follicles with a tendency to goiter formation. Propranolol is a β-adrenergic blocking agent used in the treatment of thyrotoxicosis (e.g., tachycardia, tremor, sweating, heat intolerance, and anxiety), but it is not goitrogenic.

118. The answer is C (2, 4). (*Biochemistry, 2nd ed, Chapter 15 II B 1 a; Chapter 31 IV A 1, 5 b, F 4; Table 31-1*) Severe dietary deficiency of thiamine (vitamin B_1) causes beriberi, the Sinhalese term for "weakness," and in alcoholics, Wernicke's encephalopathy. The cardiac disease of beriberi is characterized by an enlargement, usually dilatation, of the heart, absence of arrhythmia, predominant failure of the right ventricle, bounding arterial pulsations, and a high-output failure. The manifestations of polyneuropathy include weakness, paresthesias, and sometimes pain. The ocular disturbances consist of weakness or paralysis (ophthalmoplegia) of the external recti, nystagmus, and palsies of conjugate gaze. The majority of patients are apathetic, listless, and severely confused. Diarrhea and dermatitis are associated with pellagra, which is due to a deficiency of nicotinic acid (niacin).

119. The answer is B (1, 3). (*Biochemistry, 2nd ed, Chapter 16 VIII D 3 b; Obstetrics and Gynecology Chapter 15 II E; Table 15-2; Pharmacology, 2nd ed, Chapter 7 III B 1, 2, 6 a, 7 e; Surgery Chapter 13 VIII D 1*) Warfarin, the drug of choice among oral anticoagulants, is a coumarin derivative that is used to prevent coagulation of blood only in vivo. Its mechanism of action is to prevent the hepatic synthesis of the active forms of vitamin K–dependent clotting factors, such as prothrombin (factor II) and factors VII, IX, and X. Thus, warfarin depresses prothrombin activity and is a vitamin K antagonist. If administered during pregnancy, warfarin can cause fetal bone abnormalities. This compound is used as a rodenticide because it produces fatal internal hemorrhage in rats.

120. The answer is C (2, 4). (*Physiology Chapter 7 VI H 1 a, b; VII F 1 a; X C 1 d, E 1 a*) Glucagon stimulates glycogenolysis in liver and epinephrine promotes glycogenolysis in muscle and liver. Glycogenolysis in liver results in the secretion of glucose because the liver (and kidney) contains the enzyme glucose-6-phosphatase, which is not present in muscle. Muscle glycogenolysis results in the elevation of blood lactate, which serves as a gluconeogenic substrate that is converted to glucose in the liver. Insulin and cortisol promote glycogenesis. Both glucagon and epinephrine are gluconeogenic hormones.

121. The answer is A (1, 2, 3). (*Physiology Chapter 1 III B*) All preganglionic neurons are cholinergic, including those that innervate the adrenal medulla, as are the postganglionic parasympathetic fibers. The majority of postganglionic sympathetic neurons are adrenergic (i.e., they release norepinephrine); however, there are some important postganglionic sympathetic cholinergic neurons, which innervate the sweat glands (sudomotor) and blood vessels (vasomotor) in skeletal muscle.

122–126. The answers are: 122-B, 123-A, 124-A, 125-D, 126-A. (*Pathology Chapter 6 IV G 2; Chapter*

16 II D 2 b) Histoplasmosis is a fungal infection caused by a small yeast, *Histoplasma capsulatum*, that most commonly produces pulmonary disease. Infection may be asymptomatic, subclinical, and self-limited; scarred, calcified granulomas occur in healthy individuals. However, if the infection persists, it is best treated with amphotericin B.

Toxoplasmosis is a protozoan infection (*Toxoplasma gondii*) that occurs primarily as a congenital infection. Common sequelae are hydrocephalus, cerebral calcification, retinochoroiditis, convulsions, and ocular palsies. Toxoplasmosis in adults can be treated with pyrimethamine in combination with sulfonamides; however, most affected infants die within a few days or a few months, and those that live have the above-mentioned defects due to neural destruction.

127–133. The answers are: 127-A, 128-B, 129-D, 130-A, 131-C, 132-B, 133-D. [*Biochemistry, 2nd ed, Chapter 27 IV A 1; Chapter 31 II A 5, B 5, D 5, F 4; Medicine Chapter 3 I B 3 a (1); Pathology Chapter 16 II E 1; Chapter 17 II A 3 b (1) (c); Pediatrics Chapter 13 III D 1 b (2)*] Pellagra, a disease affecting the skin (dermatitis), the gastrointestinal tract (diarrhea), and the central nervous system (dementia), is the result of a niacin deficiency. Because niacin can be formed from tryptophan, an essential amino acid, dietary treatment of pellagra must take into consideration daily allowances of niacin and tryptophan. Endemic pellagra is no longer a common occurrence; however, it is a manifestation of two disorders of tryptophan metabolism, Hartnup disease and the carcinoid syndrome. Hartnup disease is an autosomal recessive defect in which patients have a reduced ability to convert tryptophan to niacin. In the carcinoid syndrome, dietary tryptophan is metabolized in the hydroxylation pathway (a minor pathway), leaving little tryptophan for the formation of niacin. Administration of large amounts of niacin can cure the pellagra associated with these conditions.

Beriberi is a severe thiamine deficiency syndrome associated with malnutrition, which is endemic to areas where there is a high intake of highly milled (polished) rice. Clinical characteristics of this deficiency range from cardiovascular and neurologic lesions to emotional disturbances. Cardiovascular changes include right-sided enlargement (dilatation), tachycardia, and "high output" cardiac failure. Neuromuscular manifestations include peripheral neuropathy (neuritis), weakness, fatigue, and an impaired capacity to work. Edema and anorexia are also characteristic. In the United States, thiamine deficiency is seen primarily in association with chronic alcoholism, which leads to Wernicke's encephalopathy, which presents with the classic triad of confusion, ataxia, and ophthalmoplegia. In thiamine deficiency, motor and sensory peripheral nerve lesions are marked by neuromuscular findings of numbness and tingling of the legs, and atrophy and weakness of the muscles of the extremities compounded by the loss of reflexes. Mental depression may also accompany these findings. The dementia caused by niacin deficiency results from degeneration of the ganglion cells of the brain, accompanied by degeneration of the fibers of the spinal cord. In the United States, the groups most likely to develop thiamine deficiency are the lower income groups (i.e., the elderly and welfare recipients), food faddists, and particularly, chronic alcoholics with their restricted dietary habits.

The most characteristic sign of ariboflavinosis is cheilitis, or angular stomatitis (i.e., fissuring at the corners of the mouth). Correlates of riboflavin deficiency also include glossitis, hyperkeratosis of the epidermis, local ulceration, and proliferation of corneal capillaries.

Pernicious anemia, a megaloblastic anemia, is the classic consequence of vitamin B_{12} (cobalamin) deficiency. In contrast to the other water-soluble vitamins, significant amounts of vitamin B_{12} are stored in the body (liver), and, therefore, it may take several years for the characteristics of B_{12} deficiency to become clinically manifested. Vitamin B_{12} deficiency is rarely due to lack of the vitamin in the diet, but rather to a failure to absorb the vitamin from the intestine. Thus, the deficiency may develop in individuals who have undergone partial or total gastrectomy or ileal resection.

134–138. The answers are: 134-A, 135-A, 136-B, 137-C, 138-A. (*Histology and Embryology Chapter 24 B 1, 2*) The light-sensitive receptors of the retina consist of millions of minute cells called rods and cones. The rods distinguish only the white and the black aspects of an image, while the cones can distinguish colors as well. The central part of the retina called the fovea centralis has only cones, which allow this portion to have very sharp vision, while only a diffuse type of vision is mediated by the rods, which are situated more at the periphery. The retina contains large quantities of the photoreactive substances, rhodopsin (in the rods) and iodopsin (in the cones). Rhodopsin is an unstable compound, which lasts only a fraction of a second in the rods; after a chemical reaction, it breaks down to retinene and scotopsin. The chemical reaction initiates impulses from the retina to the optic nerve.

139–143. The answers are: 139-A, 140-B, 141-D, 142-B, 143-D. (*Immunology Chapter 7 IV A; Microbiology Chapter 10 II B*) Tetanus immunizations are compulsory for children in the United States as tetanus can be prevented by the regular administration of tetanus toxoid. This toxoid is prepared by chemical denaturation of active neurotoxin that is isolated from culture filtrates. The toxoid includes immunoglobulin (antibody) production that is capable of inactivating toxin released by *Clostridium tetani*. Neither tetanus toxoid nor tetanus antitoxin leads to the production of antibodies against *C. tetani* nor has any bactericidal activity against *C. tetani*. Primary immunization against tetanus with adsorbed toxoid is superior to giving antitoxin at the time of injury to a previously immunized patient. An inadequately immunized patient should be given tetanus immune globulin (human). The benefit of the antiserum depends on how much tetanospasmin is already bound to the synaptic membranes. Antitoxin of animal origin (made from horse or bovine serum) is far less preferable because there is considerable risk of serum sickness. Serum sickness is an allergic reaction following the administration of a foreign substance (e.g., horse serum) or certain drugs (e.g., penicillin) characterized by fever, arthralgias, skin rash, and lymphadenopathy.

144–148. The answers are: 144-A, 145-A, 146-B, 147-C, 148-D. [*Biochemistry, 2nd ed, Chapter 31 III A 4 a, b, 5 a, B; Medicine Chapter 3 V D 2 a; Chapter 9 VIII A 1, 2; Pathology Chapter 17 III B 2 a; Chapter 19 I E 1–3; Pediatrics Chapter 13 VI F 3 a–c; Chapter 15 VII B 2 a (1); Pharmacology, 2nd ed, Chapter 7 III B 1–3; Physiology Chapter 1 IX A 2 b (2)*] Vitamin A consists of three biologically active forms: retinol, retinal, and retinoic acid. Like all fat-soluble vitamins, it is stored throughout the body but primarily in the liver. Clinical manifestations of vitamin A deficiency include nyctalopia (nightblindness). Impairment of visual acuity in dim light is usually the first demonstrable change in hypovitaminosis A. A severe deficiency of this vitamin can lead to keratinization of the limbal conjunctiva (xerophthalmia). Vitamin A is a component of visual pigment, rhodopsin.

In hypovitaminosis A, there is a cessation of bone remodeling with the loss of osteoclastic activity. The bones are short and thick with a predominance of new cancellous periosteum. In hypervitaminosis A, there is abundant mineralization of the periosteum and abnormal bone formation. Liver, kidney, cream, butter, and egg yolks are good sources of preformed vitamin A, while yellow and green vegetables and fruits are good dietary sources of carotenes, which are precursors of vitamin A.

In adults, whose bony growth is complete, bone deformities are rare with a vitamin D deficiency. However, in hypovitaminosis D in adults, there is an increased radiolucency of bones and an increased tendency for fractures to occur. This condition is called osteomalacia, or adult rickets. In vitamin C deficiency, there is a decrease in the trabecular bone mass and the osteoblasts are abnormal. Natural sources of preformed vitamin D are ergocalciferol (vitamin D_2) found in plants and cholecalciferol (vitamin D_3) found in animal tissues. Vitamins D_2 and D_3 become biologically active in vivo by two hydroxylation reactions. Vitamin D occurs naturally in fatty fish, eggs, liver, and butter. Milk fortified with vitamin D is a good dietary source.

Vitamin K is required for the hepatic synthesis of prothrombin and the blood clotting factors II, VII, IX, and X. A deficiency of this vitamin in adults is unlikely because it is synthesized by intestinal bacteria and it is widely distributed in food. A prolonged coagulation (prothrombin) time is characteristic of vitamin K deficiency, which is sometimes observed in neonates. Coagulopathies can occur with liver failure, nutritional deficiency of vitamin K, malabsorption, and through drug therapy (e.g., antibiotics, which reduce intestinal flora, and vitamin K antagonists, such as coumarin, warfarin, and heparin).

149–154. The answers are: 149-B, 150-D, 151-E, 152-D, 153-E, 154-B. [*Biochemistry, 2nd ed, Chapter 10 I C 2 b, c (1); Chapter 11 IV C 2 a; V A 1, B 2, C 2; VIII A, H; Physiology Chapter 3 II C 1*] The velocity of an enzyme reaction increases with substrate concentration until a maximal velocity (V_{max}) is attained. Curve B is a rectangular hyperbola showing the relationship between velocity and substrate concentration.

An inhibitor is a substance that decreases the velocity of an enzyme-catalyzed reaction. When an inhibitor binds reversibly to the same site as the substrate, it competes with the substrate for that site (competitive inhibition). The reaction velocity reaches the V_{max} observed without inhibitor when the substrate concentration is sufficiently high. When an inhibitor and substrate bind at different sites on the enzyme, it is called noncompetitive inhibition. The inhibitor can bind to the enzyme or the enzyme–substrate complex, reducing the reaction velocity. Increasing substrate concentration does not reverse the effect of noncompetitive inhibition, and, therefore, V_{max} decreases. Curve D shows the inhibitory effect of excess substrate on enzyme reaction velocity.

Curve E summarizes the effects of an enzyme modifier that enhances the enzyme reaction and is called a positive modifier. Allosteric enzymes are regulated by substances called effectors (modifiers) that bind noncovalently at a site other than the active site. If the presence of the substrate on one site influences the binding of substrate to vacant sites or influences the rate of product formation at other occupied sites, then the substrate itself acts as a modifier, causing substrate activation or substrate inhibition. Generally, allosteric enzymes yield sigmoidal velocity curves. Curve A cannot be a logical choice because there is a high reaction rate in the absence of substrate.

Curve D is a bell-shaped curve that shows the effect of changes in pH on the rate of an enzyme-catalyzed reaction. Curve D indicates that there is an optimal pH for the activity of an enzyme.

The oxygen association–dissociation curve for hemoglobin (curve E) is sigmoidal in shape (see the figure on the next page). The reason that the curve is S-shaped and not linear is that it is actually a plot of four reactions rather than one. Thus, each of the four heme-containing subunits of hemoglobin can combine with one molecule of oxygen.

The oxygen association–dissociation curve for myoglobin (curve B) has a hyperbolic shape. Myoglobin has a higher oxygen affinity than hemoglobin and, therefore, is shifted to the left. Thus, the partial pressure of oxygen (PO_2) required to attain half-saturation of the binding sites (P_{50}) is much less. The O_2 affinity and the P_{50} are inversely related, and, therefore, the more tightly oxygen binds, the lower is the P_{50}.

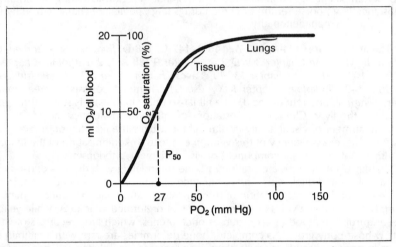

Reprinted with permission from Bullock J, et al: *Physiology*. Media, PA, Harwal, 1984, p 142.

155–159. The answers are: 155-D, 156-E, 157-B, 158-C, 159-A. [*Pharmacology, 2nd ed, Chapter 2 I F 2; III A 3 a (2); VII C 1; Table 2-3; Chapter 5 I C 3 c; IV B 3, F 2 a, c, I 1 a (1)–(3), d (1) (a) (i), 2 b; Chapter 6 IX A 1 a, c, 2; Chapter 8 V C 1 a–c, 2 a–d*] Triamterene, an orally active potassium-sparing diuretic that does not require the presence of endogenous aldosterone or any other mineralocorticoid, is used in combination with other diuretics for the treatment of hypertension. It is an orally active pteridine that produces natriuresis by decreasing sodium ion (Na^+) reabsorption in the distal tubule that is independent of aldosterone. The decrease in distal tubular Na^+ reabsorption produces a drop in the availability of Na^+ to the Na^+-K^+ exchange pump with a resultant decline in Na^+ reabsorption and, therefore, a reduced secretion of potassium ion (K^+). Additionally, triamterene inhibits hydrogen ion (H^+) secretion in the distal tubule and collecting duct. This diuretic is clinically useful in the treatment of edema.

Captopril, an antagonist of the renin–angiotensin–aldosterone system, is a specific competitive inhibitor of pulmonary peptidyl dipeptidase (angiotensin-converting enzyme), which converts angiotensin I to angiotensin II. The reduction in angiotensin II leads to a decline in aldosterone secretion and, in turn, a decline in Na^+ and water retention and a decline in K^+ secretion. Captopril, when administered orally, will reduce blood pressure in hypertensive patients regardless of the plasma renin levels. Because the angiotensin-converting enzyme is also known as kininase II, which is necessary for the inactivation of bradykinin, captopril may increase the concentration of bradykinin, which is a potent vasodilator.

Trimethaphan, a ganglionic nicotinic blocking agent, acts as a competitive acetylcholine antagonist and competes with this neurotransmitter for nicotinic receptors on autonomic postsynaptic ganglia, thereby blocking transmission. It is used therapeutically in treating hypertensive crises, in the management of autonomic hyperreflexia, and to provide controlled hypotension in order to reduce bleeding in the operative field during surgery.

Saralasin, an angiotensin II analogue, is a competitive inhibitor of angiotensin II receptors. It has been shown to have an antihypertensive effect in patients with renovascular hypertension, end-stage renal disease, high-renin essential hypertension, and malignant hypertension following intravenous administration. This drug is a diagnostic aid in the identification of patients with angiotensin-dependent hypertension (i.e., in the detection of patients with renovascular hypertension).

Prazosin is selective for α_1 receptors [i.e., it preferentially blocks responses mediated by the postsynaptic α receptors in the blood vessels (α_1)]. Given orally, this antihypertensive drug causes vasodilation primarily in arterial smooth muscle. The antihypertensive action of prazosin is potentiated by the coadministration of thiazide diuretics. Since it does not significantly influence blood uric acid or glucose levels, it can be used in hypertensive patients whose condition is complicated by diabetes mellitus or gout.

160–164. The answers are: 160-A, 161-B, 162-C, 163-D, 164-E. (*Anatomy Chapter 29 VII B 4; Tables 29-5 and 29-10*) The circle of Willis, located beneath the hypothalamus and surrounding the optic chiasm and the pituitary stalk, is composed of a vascular ring formed by the anastomoses between branches of the internal carotid arteries anteriorly and branches of the vertebral arteries posteriorly. The anterior part of the brain is perfused with blood from the internal carotids through the anterior and middle cerebral arteries; the brain stem, cerebellum, and parts of the temporal and occipital lobes are supplied by the vertebral arteries. The vessels that form the anastomoses that make up the circle are the single anterior communicating artery, which connects the left and right anterior circulations, and the two posterior communicating arteries. The components of the circle are the single anterior communicating artery and the paired anterior cerebral, internal carotid, posterior communicating, and posterior cerebral arteries. The superior, anterior–inferior, and posterior–inferior cerebellar arteries perfuse the cerebellum and parts of the brain stem. In patients with coarctation of the aorta, the vessels of the circle of Willis are prone to the formation of berry aneurysms, which may rupture, causing a subarachnoid hemorrhage. See the figure below.

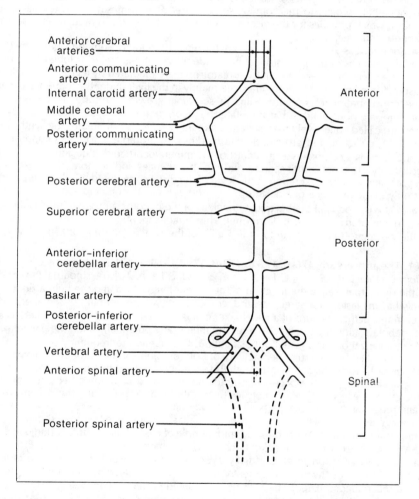

165–169. The answers are: 165-A, 166-D, 167-C, 168-E, 169-B. [*Microbiology Chapter 10 II B, D; Chapter 11 II C 1 b; Chapter 13 I E; Chapter 15 I G 1 a (1)*] *Clostridium novyi* is the etiologic agent in gas gangrene. It is prevalent in the soil. Serotypes A and B produce an alpha toxin that is lethal and causes increased capillary permeability.

Vibrio cholerae is the etiologic agent of cholera, a diarrhea syndrome known as ''rice-water'' stools, that can be fatal. Cholera is spread by the ingestion of fecally contaminated food and water. This disease is prevalent in the Far East, India, Middle East, and Africa.

Treponema vincentii is the etiologic agent of acute necrotizing ulcerative gingivitis, or trench mouth, when it grows in combination with *Bacteroides melaninogenicus*. The disease may actually be caused by a herpesvirus that promotes the overgrowth of the two above-mentioned bacteria.

Chlamydia trachomatis (serotypes A, B, Ba, and C) is the etiologic agent of trachoma. Infection is usually acquired in infancy as acute conjunctivitis and is a leading cause of blindness. Approximately 400 million people worldwide have trachoma, and of these, 20 million are blind.

Clostridium tetani is the etiologic agent of tetanus, also known as lockjaw. This condition is caused by a neurotoxic exotoxin (tetanospasmin) that results in peripheral nerve and muscle spasms. Spasm of the masseters accounts for the name "lockjaw."

170–175. The answers are: 170-E, 171-D, 172-C, 173-B, 174-A, 175-D. [*Biochemistry, 2nd ed, Chapter 30 I B 3 d; Histology and Embryology Chapter 16 V B 2 c; Chapter 20 V B 3 d (2), (3); Pediatrics Chapter 15 IV A 1; Pharmacology, 2nd ed, Chapter 5 IV B 3; Chapter 6 IX B 1, 2; Physiology Chapter 4 IX F 1, 2; Chapter 7 V D 1 b–d*] The somesthetic cortex is a primary area of the cerebral cortex responsible for the perception of somatosensory information conveyed via the ascending (sensory) pathways from cutaneous, muscle, tendon, and joint receptors. It is also referred to as the sensory cortex, which is located on the postcentral gyrus of the parietal lobe. Input from touch, pressure, pain, temperature, and proprioceptors project to this somatic sensory area. The somesthetic cortex has a somatotopic organization, which provides for the discrete localization of the various modalities of sensation from a distinct peripheral area.

Growth hormone is also referred to as somatotropic hormone or somatotropin, which is produced by the acidophil cells of the pars distalis of the adenohypophysis (anterior lobe of the pituitary).

Many of the effects on linear growth by somatotropin are mediated by a group of insulin-like growth factors (somatomedins), which are synthesized mainly in the liver under the influence of somatotropin; thus, the concentration of somatomedins in serum is growth hormone–dependent. Because the somatomedins are polypeptides that stimulate the incorporation of sulfate into proteoglycans of cartilage, they are called collectively the "sulfation factor," which also stimulates the synthesis in cartilage of RNA, DNA, collagen, and protein. Somatomedins also promote mitosis of chondrocytes.

Spironolactone is a competitive antagonist of the mineralocorticoid, aldosterone. It is an antihypertensive drug that is a potassium-sparing diuretic. It enhances sodium ion (Na^+) excretion and decreases potassium ion (K^+) excretion at the level of the distal convoluted tubule. This antagonist is efficacious only in the presence of aldosterone or another mineralocorticoid.

Somatostatin is produced by the arcuate nucleus of the hypothalamus and inhibits the synthesis and secretion of somatotropin (growth hormone). This tetradecapeptide is also found in other parts of the brain, the gastrointestinal tract, and in the δ cells of the pancreatic islets of Langerhans.

176–181. The answers are: 176-B, 177-B, 178-B, 179-C, 180-A, 181-D. [*Anatomy Chapter 13 VII A 1 a; Physiology Chapter 2 II B 3 c (5), C 1, 4 a (2) (a), 5 c; VII B 1 a, b, 2 a*] The sinoatrial (SA) node is embedded in the right atrial wall at the junction of the superior vena cava and the right atrium. The SA node ordinarily has the fastest discharge rate and, consequently, is the normal "pacemaker." The principal distinguishing electrical feature of a pacemaker cell is found in phase 4 in which there is a slow spontaneous depolarization (i.e., decrease in resting membrane potential) called the pacemaker potential, diastolic depolarization, or phase 4 depolarization. Ordinarily, the frequency of pacemaker depolarization is controlled by the integrated activity of both divisions of the autonomic nervous system. Increased sympathetic neural activity, through the secretion of norepinephrine, increases the heart rate by increasing the slope of the pacemaker potential. Increased parasympathetic activity, through the vagal secretion of acetylcholine, diminishes heart rate by hyperpolarizing the pacemaker cell membrane and reducing the slope of the pacemaker potential.

The average inherent discharge rates of the specialized conductive tissues of the heart are: SA node = 72/min; atrioventricular (AV) node = 60/min; bundle of His = 50/min; and Purkinje fibers = 30/min.

The SA node is the cardiac pacemaker because its cells have the steepest phase 4. From the SA node, the wave of depolarization spreads radially over the atrial myocardium and more rapidly over the specialized atrial conductive fibers to the AV node. Atrial depolarization inscribes the P wave on the scalar electrocardiogram (ECG). The AV node is situated posteriorly on the right side of the interatrial septum near the ostium of the coronary sinus. An important characteristic of the AV node is its very low conduction velocity, allowing for the delay between atrial and ventricular activation. The excitation process then is conducted rapidly down the common bundle of His with its left and right branches on either side of the interventricular septum to the Purkinje network, causing the ventricles to be depolarized from the endocardial surface to the epicardial surface. Ventricular depolarization inscribes the QRS complex on the scalar electrocardiogram. The conduction velocity of the action potential over the Purkinje fiber system is the fastest of any tissue within the heart, reaching a speed of about 4 m/sec.

Afferent fibers from baroreceptors in the walls of the aortic arch and carotid sinus travel via the aortic and carotid sinus nerves, join the vagus and glossopharyngeal nerves, respectively, and make connections with the cardiovascular centers in the medulla. The stretching of these baroreceptors generates action potentials in these afferent nerves whose frequency is proportional to the pressure change within the artery. Thus, increased arterial pressure at the baroreceptor site will increase the frequency of firing along these sensory nerves, resulting in an inhibition of the pressor area (i.e., a decrease in sympathetic tone) and facilitation of the depressor area (i.e., an increase in parasympathetic tone). The result of this increase in blood pressure is a decrease in heart rate (bradycardia) and blood pressure (vasodilation).

182–186. The answers are: 182-B, 183-D, 184-C, 185-E, 186-A. [*Biochemistry, 2nd ed, Chapter 20 VI B 4; Chapter 23 IV B 3; Chapter 27 II C 2 e; IV A 1; Chapter 29 VII A 2 a; Chapter 31 II A 1–5, D, F; III A 5, B; Medicine Chapter 3 I B 3 a; Chapter 6 XIV B 5*] Nicotinic acid (niacin) is the main, but not the sole, dietary defect in pellagra. Low tryptophan also plays a role because dietary tryptophan is a source of niacin. Hartnup disease patients have a reduced ability to convert tryptophan to niacin, which results in pellagra. Late manifestations of niacin deficiency include diarrhea, dermatitis, and depression.

Thiamine hydrochloride (vitamin B_1) deficiency results in beriberi, late manifestations of which include anorexia, polyneuritis, serous effusions, and high output cardiac failure. Cardiac problems are associated with severe beriberi, including right-sided enlargement, tachycardia, and cardiac failure. Wernicke's encephalopathy is the result of an acute thiamine deficiency seen primarily in alcoholics.

Vitamin B_{12} (cobalamin) deficiency as a result of an absorption defect can cause pernicious anemia. Predisposition to pernicious anemia is probably inherited as an autosomal dominant trait where there is a deficiency of intrinsic factor, a glycoprotein produced by the gastric parietal cells, which is necessary for the ileal absorption of vitamin B_{12}. Clinical vitamin B_{12} deficiency may also be caused by gastrectomy, regional ileitis, resection of the ileum, and fish tapeworm disease. Pernicious anemia appears when the body's vitamin B_{12} pool has been reduced to 10% of normal. The hepatic biologic half-life of vitamin B_{12} is between 2 and 5 years.

Vitamin D_3 (cholecalciferol) taken in excessive amounts is the most toxic of all vitamins. It can result in increased serum calcium and inorganic phosphate, resulting in metastatic calcification of soft tissue (e.g., nephrocalcinosis and calcium deposition in the arteries).

Hypovitaminosis A may cause dry skin, tunnel vision, night blindness, and follicular hyperkeratosis.

187–190. The answers are: 187-D, 188-A, 189-B, 190-C. (*Preventive Medicine and Public Health Chapter 3 I C 1, 2*) Distribution is the summary of the frequency of a characteristic for a series of data from a sample or population. A "bell-shaped" curve is normal and anything that diverges from a symmetrical bell-shaped distribution is abnormal. All of the other diagrams in the question depict irregular distribution curves. A bimodal distribution is the occurrence of two frequency peaks of a characteristic for a series of data. Skewed distributions are those that are asymmetric, and they are named according to their "tail." If the tail is among the higher values being characterized, the distribution is skewed to the right or positively skewed.

191–196. The answers are: 191-B, 192-C, 193-A, 194-D, 195-E, 196-C. [*Pharmacology, 2nd ed, Chapter 2 IV B 1, G 1; V A 1, 2, 4 a (1); VI A 1, 4 b; VIII A 1 a, C 1 a; Chapter 8 V E 1 b (1)*] Methacholine, a methyl derivative of acetylcholine, is a cholinomimetic drug, which has pharmacologic effects identical to those obtained with acetylcholine. Thus, it elicits vasodilation, bradycardia (negative chronotropism), a decrease in the force of myocardial contraction (negative inotropism), and increased gastrointestinal motility and secretion; it causes smooth muscle contraction in the uterus, ureters, bladder (detrusor muscle), bronchioles, and pupillary sphincter muscle (miosis). Acetylcholine and methacholine are hydrolyzed by acetylcholinesterase. *In contrast to acetylcholine, methacholine exerts essentially no nicotinic effects.* With regard to muscarinic effects, methacholine mimics the activity of acetylcholine. Methacholine still retains its usefulness as a diagnostic tool in cases of suspected poisoning due to atropine or other belladonna alkaloids. The diagnosis is confirmed by the failure of subcutaneously injected methacholine to elicit characteristic signs of flush, salivation, lacrimation, and enhanced gastrointestinal motility.

Physostigmine (eserine) is a tertiary amine and a carbamate anticholinesterase, which inhibits acetylcholinesterase by binding to it covalently. Thus, the pharmacologic properties of physostigmine mimic those of acetylcholine. Anticholinesterase drugs are used to enhance neuromuscular transmission in some conditions, such as myasthenia gravis, because they prolong the action of endogenous acetylcholine by inhibiting the enzyme acetylcholinesterase. Excessive doses may impair neuromuscular transmission by causing a depolarization block. Many of the peripheral and central nevous system effects of atropine poisoning and related anticholinergics can be reversed by the intravenous injection of physostigmine salicylate. This drug is now mainly used as a miotic.

Atropine, a muscarinic blocker, is an anticholinergic tertiary amine that exerts its effect through the competitive antagonism of acetylcholine by binding to muscarinic receptors of peripheral tissue and in the central nervous system. All postganglionic parasympathetic fibers and those postganglionic sympathetic fibers that release acetylcholine as a neurotransmitter (cholinergic sympathetic fibers) form synapses on tissues that contain muscarinic receptors. At the neuromuscular junction and adrenal medulla, nicotinic receptors are the mediators of acetylcholine responses, and muscarinic blocking agents are without effect at those sites. This tertiary amine is used as an anticholinergic premedication (preanesthetic) drug to dry bronchial and salivary secretions, which are increased by intubation and the inhalational anesthetics. It is also used to prevent excessive bradycardia and hypotension caused by other drugs (i.e., halothane, thiopental, succinylcholine, and neostigmine).

Succinylcholine, a dicholine ester that is rapidly hydrolyzed by plasma acetylcholinesterase, mimics the action of acetylcholine at the skeletal muscle neuromuscular junction. Succinylcholine maintains the muscle in a depolarized state for the duration of the drug infusion. Thus, following an initial stimulation of skeletal muscles, it results in transmission failure and muscle relaxation. This effect of succinylcholine provides a controlled muscle paralysis during surgery. Succinylcholine has little effect on autonomic ganglia or postganglionic cholinergic neurons. The duration of action of this depolarizing muscle relaxant is prolonged because its dissociation from the receptor site and enzymatic hydrolysis is slower than acetylcholine.

No known substances interfere with the storage of acetylcholine; however, the toxin of the microorganism *Clostridium botulinum* interferes with the *release* of acetylcholine. By inhibiting the release of acetylcholine, the botulinum toxin inhibits cholinergic transmission to the skeletal muscles controlling respiration, and death follows from asphyxiation. Botulism occurs most commonly as a result of faulty sterilization of home-canned foods.

197–201. The answers are: 197-D, 198-A, 199-E, 200-B, 201-C. (*Pharmacology, 2nd ed, Chapter 3 IV D 1; Chapter 7 III D 2; Chapter 10 I D 1; II E 1; VI B 1 a, 2 b; VII A 3 a–c*) Metyrapone exerts its primary pharmacologic effect by inhibiting 11β-hydroxylase, thus causing a decline in the synthesis and secretion of cortisol by the adrenal cortex. When this cortisol-forming enzyme is blocked, the adrenal cortex responds by secreting higher amounts of 11-deoxycortisol, which, like cortisol, is a 17-hydroxycorticosteroid. It is employed in the differential diagnosis of primary and secondary adrenal insufficiency. When cortisol secretion is blocked, the reduction in negative feedback should increase adrenocorticotropic hormone and the secretion of cortisol precursors if the pituitary–adrenocortical axis is functional. Metyrapone has also been used to treat hypercortisolism caused by inoperable bronchogenic carcinomas or adrenal tumors.

Bromocriptine, an ergot alkaloid derivative, is a dopaminergic agonist used in the treatment of Parkinson's disease. In normal subjects, it stimulates the secretion of growth hormone (GH), while in patients with acromegaly, it paradoxically lowers the plasma concentration of GH. Bromocriptine is also effective in treating hyperprolactinemia, which often is the cause of galactorrhea, by the suppression of pituitary prolactin secretion. Hyperprolactinemia is a common cause of gonadal dysfunction: infertility, amenorrhea, or menstrual disorders in women and impotence in men.

The antithyroid drug, methimazole, is a thionamide derivative used to treat hyperthyroidism by inhibiting the incorporation of iodide into thyroglobulin to form thyroid hormone. It does not inhibit the peripheral monodeiodination of thyroxine to triiodothyronine. In usual doses, methimazole does not inactivate or interfere with the release of thyroid hormone previously formed or stored in the gland.

Danazol, a derivative of 17-ethynyl testosterone, is a weak protein anabolic agent that has important antigonadotropic properties in that it suppresses luteinizing hormone (LH) and follicle-stimulating hormone (FSH) secretion from the pituitary. The subsequent diminution in ovarian steroidogenesis accounts for the efficacy of this drug in the treatment of endometriosis. Danazol is also approved for use in fibrocystic breast disease and is being investigated for the treatment of hereditary angioneurotic edema, α_1-antitrypsin deficiency, gynecomastia, and systemic lupus erythematosus.

Clomiphene citrate is a nonsteroidal antiestrogen used to treat female infertility caused by anovulation because it increases the pituitary secretion of LH and FSH. This antiestrogen prevents the binding of estradiol in the hypothalamus and in the pituitary, thereby preventing the normal feedback inhibition of estrogens on the secretion of gonadotropin-releasing hormones and gonadotropins . This results in the enhanced secretion of gonadotropins (FSH and LH), which, in turn, leads to ovarian stimulation, ovulation, and sustained function of the corpus luteum.

202–206. The answers are: 202-A, 203-B, 204-C, 205-D, 206-E. (*Histology and Embryology Chapter 24 V*) The retina of the eye has two main components, a pigmented retina and a neural retina. These two components comprise 10 layers of the retina, five of which are indicated in the photomicrograph that accompanies the question in the following order: (A) pigmented epithelium, (B) rod and cone segments, (C) ganglion cell layer, (D) layer of optic nerve fibers, and (E) inner limiting membrane. The figure below depicts the 10 layers of the retina and indicates the light path leading to retinal receptor stimulation.

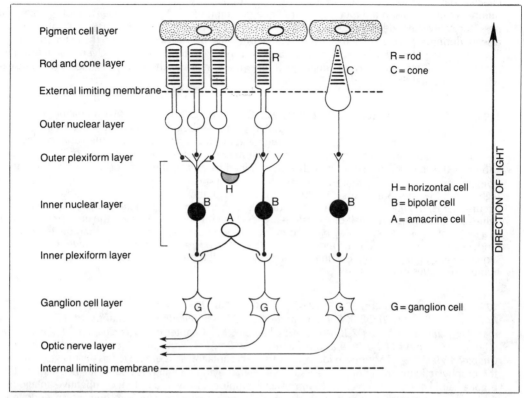

Reprinted with permission from Bullock J, et al: *Physiology*. Media, PA, Harwal, 1984, p 59.

207–213. The answers are: 207-E, 208-C, 209-C, 210-B, 211-A, 212-D, 213-C. [*Medicine Chapter 9 I A 1 a (2), b (3) (a); Physiology Chapter 1 IX F 1–4*] A complete lesion of the left optic radiation, distal to the left lateral geniculate body, interrupts fibers from the homolateral halves (left) of both retinal fields. In terms of *visual* fields, this lesion causes a loss of vision in the left nasal field and in the right temporal field with a resultant right homonymous hemianopia. Note that the condition is described as a hemianopia since one-half of the visual field is eliminated from each eye. The hemianopia is homonymous as the loss is in the same visual field (right) of each eye. These visual field defects would also occur with a complete lesion of the left optic tract.

A complete anterior–posterior lesion through the middle of the optic chiasm interrupts only the decussating fibers (i.e., those from the nasal retinas), while leaving those from the lateral (temporal) retinas intact. Because the nasal retinas are stimulated by light from the lateral (temporal) visual fields, the visual field loss is called heteronymous bitemporal hemianopia. The hemianopia is heteronymous as the visual field loss is in different halves of the two retinas. This lesion is also correctly designated as a bitemporal hemianopia. A glioma or pituitary tumor impinging on the optic chiasm is consistent with a bitemporal hemianopia.

A partial lesion at the lateral aspect of the left side of the optic chiasm interrupts uncrossed fibers emanating from the lateral half of the left retina, which is stimulated by light from the left nasal visual field. Therefore, this visual field defect is a left nasal hemianopia.

A complete section of the right optic nerve causes blindness in the right eye, that is, blindness ipsilateral to the lesion. Complete lesions of both optic tracts result in total bilateral blindness. At the optic chiasm, fibers initiating nasally cross over so that the left optic tract contains fibers from the left halves of both retinas, and the right optic tract contains fibers from corresponding right halves of each retina.

Craniopharyngiomas are probably derived from remnants of Rathke's pouch (oral ectoderm), which is the progenitor tissue for the anterior pituitary. These tumors can encroach on the optic chiasm, leading to a bitemporal hemianopia. The incipient visual loss tends to occur first in the superior temporal quadrants (quadrantanopia) and progresses to a bitemporal visual loss.

214–218. The answers are: 214-E, 215-D, 216-C, 217-B, 218-A. (*Preventive Medicine and Public Health Chapter 1 IV B 2 a, b, 3; Chapter 2 II E 4*) Validity is the true accuracy of observed experimental effects—that is, validity describes the accuracy and reliability of a test. Morbidity is the ratio of the number of ill persons to the total population of a community—that is, it is a measure of the rate of illness. Mortality is the death rate in a given population. Prevalence is the rate of *all* cases of a specified disease during a specified time in a given population. Thus, prevalence measures the extent of illness in a population. Incidence is the rate of *new* cases of a specified disease during a given time interval in a given group of persons. Thus, incidence measures the rate at which healthy people develop disease within a specified time period.

219–223. The answers are: 219-E, 220-D, 221-C, 222-B, 223-A. (*Preventive Medicine and Public Health Chapter 3 II A 1 a, 2 a, 3 a, B 1 a, 2 a*) A normal distribution is completely determined by two constants or parameters. The mean locates the center of the distribution, and the variance describes the amount of dispersion, or scatter, of individual measurements. The square root of the variance is known as the standard deviation, which is determined by adding the sums of the squared deviations from the mean and dividing that sum by the number of observations in the series minus 1. Range is the highest and lowest scores of a series. Median is the point above and below which 50% of the scores occur—that is, the median is the value that divides the series into two equal groups so that half of the values are greater than and half of the values are less than the median. Mode is the most frequent score in a series of values. A series may have no mode (i.e., no value occurring more than once) or several modes (i.e., several different frequency peaks). Mean is the arithmetic average of individual scores—that is, the mean is the value that is the sum of all the values in a series divided by the actual number of values in the series.

224–228. The answers are: 224-E, 225-D, 226-C, 227-B, 228-A. [*Medicine Chapter 4 I F 2; III E 2 c; IV E 4 a (3); VIII F 2 b (2) (b); IX G 1 b; Chapter 5 VII C 5 c–e; Microbiology Chapter 14 II E 2 a (5); Pharmacology, 2nd ed, Chapter 2 III A 4 c (4); Chapter 6 I B; Chapter 8 V B 1; Chapter 11 V B 2 a (1), b (1)–(3), 4, 6 a, c; VI D 2 a, 4, 6 a, b; Chapter 12 IX B 4, 6 a; Preventive Medicine and Public Health Chapter 4 VII C 2 a (3)*] Methysergide, an α-adrenergic antagonist, is employed as an analgesic agent for the prophylactic treatment of severe recurrent migraine and migrainous neuralgia. This semisynthetic ergot alkaloid congener, which lacks intrinsic vasomotor activity, is a potent competitive antagonist of 5-hydroxytryptamine (i.e., serotonin). Because of the possible role of serotonin as an endogenous mediator of cranial vasodilatation and because methysergide is an antiserotoninergic agent, methysergide exerts a slight vasoconstrictor effect. Chronic use of this autacoid antagonist can cause retroperitoneal fibrosis and fibrosis of the heart valves and pleura.

Ethambutol is an anti-infective agent used in combination with other agents for the treatment of tuberculosis, a disease caused by *Mycobacterium tuberculosis*, which primarily affects the lungs but also may affect the meninges, genitourinary tract, bones, and other organs. This bacteriostat has replaced para-aminosalicylic acid as a first-line drug for use in combination with rifampin and isoniazid. Although well tolerated, the major side effect of ethambutol is an optic neuritis that affects the central fibers of the optic nerve, resulting in the loss of central vision and impaired red–green discrimination. These effects may be unilateral or bilateral and are usually reversible.

Cisplatin, a novel cytotoxic drug containing platinum, has a mechanism of action analogous to the alkylating agents (e.g., cyclophosphamide). It binds adjacent guanine residues on the same DNA strand, leading to inhibition of DNA synthesis. This antineoplastic drug is one of the most effective agents in solid tumors. In combination with bleomycin and vinblastine, cisplatin produces cures in the majority of patients with metastatic testicular cancer, as well as germ cell cancers of the ovary. It is a major agent in combination chemotherapy for ovarian adenocarcinomas. Common toxicity problems include nephrotoxicity, ototoxicity (e.g., high-tone hearing loss and tinnitus), and peripheral neuropathy. Creatinine clearance should be closely monitored because of the nephrotoxicity.

Streptozocin (streptozotocin) is a glycosylated nitrosourea (i.e., alkylating antineoplastic drug) because it acts by methylation of nucleic acids. Its cytotoxic action includes the rapid and severe depletion of the pyridine nucleotides, nicotinamide-adenine dinucleotide (NAD^+) and reduced NAD^+ (NADH), in the liver and pancreatic islets. As an anticancer drug, it is associated with a high remission rate in patients with islet carcinomas of the pancreas. It is also useful in malignant carcinoid tumors. The major toxicity of this antitumor agent is renal tubular damage, with pathologic correlates of proteinuria, hypophosphatemia, aminoacidemia, and renal tubular acidosis.

Tamoxifen is a synthetic nonsteroidal antiestrogen used as an antineoplastic agent in the treatment of postmenopausal metastatic breast carcinoma. This hormone antagonist avidly binds to cytoplasmic estrogen receptors within target cells and competes with endogenous estrogens for these receptor sites. Adverse reactions with this anticancer drug include hot flashes, bone pain, and hypercalcemia.

229–233. The answers are: 229-E, 230-B, 231-C, 232-D, 233-A. (*Biochemistry, 2nd ed, Chapter 22 IV C 2 c; Medicine Chapter 10 III H 3 a (2) (a) (ii); V G 2 a (1) (b); Pharmacology, 2nd ed, Chapter 3 IX F 4; Chapter 9 II F 4; Chapter 14 III B 2 g, 3 e, 4 e, 6 a (1), b, d; Pediatrics Chapter 2 IX F 1 d, 2 b (5), 4 d (2); Chapter 4 VII H 3; Preventive Medicine and Public Health Chapter 12 IV A 1, 4 d (3), 5; Psychiatry Chapter 3 IV G 3; Chapter 4 II E 3*] Naloxone, a pure opioid antagonist, is usually administered parenterally to reverse within 1–2 min the sedative effects, respiratory depression, and untoward cardiovascular effects caused by narcotic (e.g., morphine sulfate) overdosage.

Dimercaprol (British antilewisite, BAL) is a chelating agent used as an antidote for arsenic, antimony, bismuth, gold, mercury, and thallium poisoning. The adverse side effects include local pain at the site of injection, paresthesias, lacrimation, blepharospasm, apprehension, asthenia, excessive salivation, and vomiting. Many of these effects are relieved by the administration of an antihistamine.

Lead poisoning is treated with chelation therapy. A combination of calcium disodium ethylenediaminetetraacetic acid (calcium disodium edetate, $CaNa_2$ EDTA) and dimercaprol is generally more effective than the use of either alone. $CaNa_2$ EDTA is used principally for lead poisoning (plumbism) but has been used for iron, copper, and zinc poisoning as well. $CaNa_2$ EDTA, which is used as a chelating agent in severe hypercalcemia, should not be used indiscriminately in the treatment of heavy metal poisoning because it will produce severe hypocalcemia.

The term salicylism is generally applied to the characteristic symptoms, which arise from chronic salicylate therapy. These characteristics include central nervous system disturbances, such as confusion, delirium, tinnitus, dizziness, and, occasionally, psychosis. The therapeutic approach to salicylate overdosage includes three major objectives: (1) provoke emesis, if the patient is conscious, or perform gastric lavage to prevent further salicylate absorption; (2) symptomatic therapy to correct existent water or electrolyte deficits through judicious use of Ringer's solution or isotonic sodium bicarbonate; and (3) reduce tissue and serum salicylate levels through alkalinization of the urine to promote drug excretion.

Deferoxamine is a chelating agent used to treat acute iron poisoning. This substance, which has a high affinity for ferric ions, must be administered parenterally because it is poorly absorbed when taken orally.

234–239. The answers are: 234-D, 235-A, 236-E, 237-D, 238-C, 239-B. [*Pharmacology, 2nd ed, Chapter 2 I F 2; II; III A 1 a (1), B 1 c (1), C 1 a, b (1), (2), c, 2 a (1), (2), d; Table 2-3; Chapter 5 IV E 2 b (1), H 1 a, b (1), (2), d, 2 a (1) (a), d; Chapter 6 VI A 1, 3, 5, D 1, 2*] Guanethidine, an adrenergic neuron blocking drug, is one of the most potent, orally active, antihypertensive agents used in the treatment of moderate to severe hypertension. It is usually prescribed with a thiazide diuretic or together with a diuretic and a vasodilator. This sympathetic antagonist prevents the release of norepinephrine from sympathetic postganglionic neurons and also depletes these nerve endings of norepinephrine. In order for guanethidine to be effective, it must be actively taken up by these postganglionic neurons. The block of norepinephrine release explains the reduction in the contraction of vascular smooth muscle in both arteries and veins and the resultant decline in blood pressure. Parasympathetic function is not altered, a characteristic that distinguishes guanethidine from the ganglionic blocking agents. While it does not deplete catecholamines from the adrenal medulla, it may provoke the release of catecholamines from a pheochromocytoma, resulting in a hypertensive crisis. In most patients, the value of this drug is limited because it fails to control supine blood pressure without causing an unacceptable degree of postural (orthostatic) hypotension. Most of the adverse side effects of guanethidine are due to the impairment of sympathetic function and unopposed parasympathetic activity. In males, this adrenergic neuron blocking agent can be a cause of impotence and difficulty in ejaculation. Phenoxybenzamine therapy can result in retrograde ejaculation or inhibition of ejaculation.

Hydrochlorothiazide is the drug of choice in mild or moderate cardiac failure in the absence of severe pulmonary or renal failure in which there is a decreased glomerular filtration rate, increased renal sodium ion (Na^+) reabsorption, increased secretion of aldosterone, and edema. It is used in the treatment of mild essential hypertension. The antihypertensive action of the thiazides, which are also carbonic anhydrase inhibitors, is based on their ability to produce diuresis, which leads to a reduction in extracellular fluid volume. Thiazides block the proximal and distal reabsorption of Na^+. They also increase potassium ion (K^+) excretion, primarily as a consequence of increased delivery of Na^+ to the distal tubule Na^+–K^+ exchange mechanism. The hypokalemia increases the danger of digitalis toxicity in patients with heart failure and glucose intolerance. Thiazides lead to the excretion of a large urine volume, which is hyperosmotic. Another consequence of hydrochlorothiazide therapy is hyperuricemia, which can provoke a gout attack.

Both α- and β-adrenergic blockers are useful in the treatment of hypertension. Phenoxybenzamine, a long-acting, irreversible α-adrenergic antagonist, reduces systemic (and pulmonary) blood pressure by blocking vasoconstriction in both arterial and venous beds. The venous dilatory effect explains the postural hypotension, which is characteristic of α blockers. Phenoxybenzamine is not used in the routine management of essential hypertension because of its side effects. Its main use is in pheochromocytoma; it is given before and during surgery to control paroxysmal hypertension or for long-term therapy if the tumor is inoperable. The excessive secretion of catecholamines by a pheochromocytoma blocks the secretion of insulin by the stimulation of a pancreatic α-adrenergic receptor on the surface of the β cells, an effect that is reversed with phenoxybenzamine. The resultant insulin release leads to hypoglycemia.

Reserpine, unlike guanethidine, neither interferes with the release of norepinephrine in sympathetic postganglionic neurons nor the re-uptake of norepinephrine in these neurons. Instead, reserpine blocks the intraneuronal storage of norepinephrine by impairing the re-uptake of catecholamines (i.e., norepinephrine and dopamine) into the intraneuronal storage vesicles. By impairing vesicular transport of norepinephrine, it is subject to intraneuronal inactivation by monoamine oxidase. Since reserpine also blocks the vesicular uptake of dopamine, the immediate precursor of norepinephrine, the synthesis of norepinephrine declines. The combined effects of the blockade of dopamine and norepinephrine vesicular uptake lead to neurotransmitter depletion. This reserpine-induced catecholamine depletion occurs in peripheral nerves, the adrenal medulla, and the brain. However, the peripheral effects are considered to be more important in producing hypotension.

In contrast to many other antihypertensive agents, hydralazine and other vasodilators do not inhibit the activity of the sympathetic nervous system. Additionally, most vasodilators relax arterial smooth muscle to a greater extent than venous smooth muscle, thereby minimizing postural hypotension.

240–244. The answers are: 240-A, 241-B, 242-C, 243-D, 244-E. (*Biochemistry, 2nd ed, Chapter 31 II A 4, 5, C 4, 5, E 4, 5, F 3, 4; III B 3, 4*) Phosphorylation of pyridoxine yields the biologically active form of vitamin B_6. This form serves as a coenzyme for a large number of enzymes, particularly those that catalyze reactions involving amino acids, for example, transamination, deamination, decarboxylation, and condensation.

The biologically active form of folic acid is tetrahydrofolic acid. This form transfers one-carbon fragments to appropriate metabolites in the synthesis of amino acids, purines, and thymidylic acid, which is the characteristic pyrimidine of DNA.

Vitamin D_3 is converted to the active form, 1,25-dihydroxycholecalciferol, by two sequential hydroxylation reactions. The active form of vitamin D_3 stimulates the intestinal absorption of calcium and phosphate, increases the mobilization of calcium and phosphate from bone, and promotes the renal reabsorption of calcium *and* phosphate (*in physiologic amounts*).

The biologically active forms of niacin, or nicotinic acid, are nicotinamide-adenine dinucleotide (NAD^+) and nicotinamide-adenine dinucleotide phosphate ($NADP^+$). These two cofactors serve as coenzymes in oxidation–reduction reactions in which the coenzyme undergoes reduction of the pyridine ring by accepting a hydride ion (hydrogen ion plus one electron). The reduced forms of these two dinucleotides are NADH and NADPH.

Thiamine pyrophosphate is the biologically active form of the vitamin. It serves as a cofactor in the oxidative decarboxylation of keto acids. It is a cofactor in the nonoxidative reactions of the pentose phosphate pathway because it is the prosthetic group of transketolase.

245–250. The answers are: 245-B, 246-E, 247-D, 248-C, 249-A, 250-C. (*Anatomy Chapter 8 II A, B; Figure 8-1*) The radius and ulna are bones of the forearm. Because the distal shaft of the radius (A) widens transversely, it forms a major articular surface with the proximal row of carpal bones. The base of the radius contacts the scaphoid bone (C) and the lunate bone (D) to form the radiocarpal joint. Fracture of the distal radius (Colles' fracture) is only surpassed in frequency by fractures of the clavicles, ribs, and fingers. The scaphoid (navicular) bone articulates with the radius proximally, with the lunate bone medially, and with the trapezium and trapezoid bones distally. Because of its shape and location, the scaphoid is the carpal bone most prone to fracture with the risk of avascular necrosis in the proximal segment as blood vessels enter the scaphoid from the distal end. The trapezoid bone articulates with the scaphoid proximally, the trapezium laterally, the capitate and the second metacarpal medially, and the first and second metacarpals distally. The lunate bone articulates with the radius proximally, the scaphoid laterally, the triquetrum medially, and the capitate distally. Like the scaphoid bone, it transmits forces from the hand to the radius. Sesamoid bones are small nodular bones found in the tendons of the joint capsules of the hands and feet.

251. The answer is C. (*Immunology Chapter 12 IV A; V C*) A patient who has been given an incompatible blood transfusion will have a hyperacute reaction. The recipient has preformed antibodies against the blood, and as soon as the mismatched blood enters the vascular system, the antibodies begin to attack the antigen in the red blood cells, causing hemolysis. Acute rejection is a result of sensitized lymphocytes, which cause destruction of the transplanted tissue; it can take 10 to 30 days for sensitized lymphocytes to develop. Chronic rejection is associated with a slow loss of tissue function over many months and years. Graft rejection of a host occurs when an immunologically competent graft is transplanted into an immunocompromised host and the graft tissue mounts an immunologic attack on the recipient. Graft-versus-host disease primarily involves the skin, alimentary tract, and liver.

252. The answer is D. [*Preventive Medicine and Public Health Chapter 4 VIII B 3 c (2); see also Appendix for references*] Meningococcal meningitis is one of the most common types of bacterial meningitis; approximately 3000 to 4000 cases are reported each year. *Neisseria meningitidis* is the causative agent, and the mode of transmission is direct contact with the infected person. Pharyngeal carriage is high, ranging from 5% to 70%. The drug of choice is rifampin (600 mg twice daily for 2 days), which is 90% effective in terminating the carrier state; however, resistant strains can emerge in 10% of cases.

253. The answer is B. [*Pathology Chapter 20 III D 2 b (3); see also Appendix for references*] The young man in the photograph that accompanies the question is most likely to have alopecia areata, which is characterized by patchy areas of hair loss. These patchy areas may be perfectly smooth or a few hairs may be present. It often progresses to alopecia totalis or complete hair loss. Trichotillomania (i.e., a pulling out of one's hair) presents with patches of irregular hair loss; however, growing hairs are always present because they cannot be pulled out unless they are long. Male pattern baldness is the most common form of alopecia. It is characterized by thinning or absence of hair around the vertex of the scalp. There is a genetic predisposition, and it may be associated with seborrhea. The extent of the hair loss is unpredictable. Tinea capitis occurs mainly in children; it is caused by *Microsporum audouini*. It usually affects the scalp and the hair, which tends to break off. Fungal cultures should be done on involved hair and the scrapings examined using potassium hydroxide.

254. The answer is B. [*Surgery Chapter 17 II C 3 a (1)–(3)*] Coarctation of the aorta, a congenital constriction distal to the ligamentum arteriosum, is found in boys twice as often as girls. Some children are asymptomatic, while others exhibit symptoms of congestive heart failure. Physical findings include hypertension or raised blood pressure in the upper extremities; normal blood pressure but absent or diminished pulses in the lower extremities; feeble, absent, or delayed femoral pulses; and a systolic murmur.

255. The answer is B. (*Medicine Chapter 3 V A, C; Table 3-1*) Platelet function is measured by bleeding time, which is normally 2 to 7 min. If the platelet count is less than 100,000/mm³ (thrombocytopenia), bleeding time will be prolonged. Although a platelet count will not measure abnormal platelet function, thrombocytopenia indicates a need for marrow examination, which will indicate problems with platelet function.

256. The answer is B. (*Pharmacology, 2nd ed, Chapter 3 V B 3 f; Behavioral Science Chapter 2 II E 5; see also Appendix for references*) Erection, which is associated with filling of the venous sinuses, is brought about by the coupling of arteriolar dilation with venous constriction. This process is under parasympathetic control, while ejaculation is mediated by sympathetic nervous stimulation of an α_1-adrenergic mechanism. The phenothiazine antipsychotic drugs, of which chlorpromazine is a prototype, exhibit an α-adrenergic receptor blocking activity, which is thought to account for the inhibition of ejaculation in men taking chlorpromazine. Thioridazine displays a much lower degree of antiadrenergic activity than do the other phenothiazines. Thus, inhibition of ejaculation without interference with erection can be observed, especially with thioridazine.

Metoclopramide promotes gastric motility and gastric emptying and, therefore, is useful before gastric surgery or as an aid to duodenal intubation. It also has an antiemetic property, making it useful to control nausea and vomiting associated with irradiation sickness, gastritis, uremia, and gastrointestinal cancer. Propranolol is a β-adrenergic blocker. Testosterone is not useful as a treatment for premature ejaculation or even impotence unless the latter is due to hypogonadism.

257. The answer is E. (*Medicine Chapter 5 III I 1 a, b*) The Zollinger-Ellison syndrome is due to a gastrin-secreting non-β islet cell tumor. These tumors usually occur in the pancreas but may also occur in the duodenum, stomach, spleen, and lymph nodes. It may present as epigastric pain, usually due to multiple peptic ulcers that are less responsive to standard ulcer therapy. It may also present with diarrhea due to hypersecretion of gastric acid and steatorrhea resulting from damage to the intestinal mucosa, inactive pancreatic lipase, and the precipitation of bile acids. Only 10% of patients with Zollinger-Ellison syndrome have resectable lesions.

258. The answer is C. (*Pediatrics Chapter 15 V A 1, 2, 4; Figure 15-1; see also Appendix for references*) The adrenogenital syndrome associated with virilization may be caused by congenital adrenal hyperplasia, postpubertal adrenal hyperplasia, adrenal adenoma, and adrenal carcinoma. All of these conditions are associated with increased plasma and urine levels of 17-ketosteroids (e.g., dehydro-epiandrosterone, androstenedione, etiocholanolone, and androsterone) and testosterone. Congenital adrenal hyperplasia may be due to a number of enzyme deficiencies, the commonest being 21-hydroxylase and 11-hydroxylase. See the diagram below.

Cushing's syndrome is not usually associated with elevated levels of testosterone, although 17-ketosteroids are elevated. This syndrome develops due to excessive cortisol production produced either as a result of endogenous overproduction of cortisol or exogenous treatment with pharmacologic doses of cortisol for other illnesses. Although hirsutism and acne may be seen in Cushing's syndrome, there is no virilization to the degree seen with the adrenogenital syndrome.

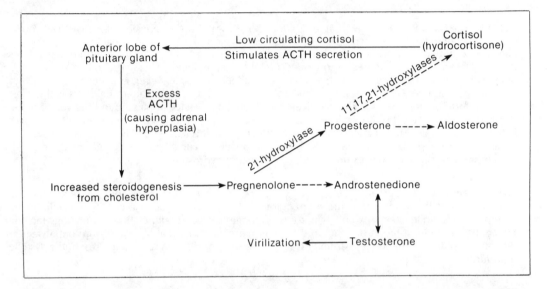

259. The answer is D. [*Medicine Chapter 9 IV A 1 b, c (3), (5), 3 c (2); Pharmacology, 2nd ed, Chapter 6 VI D 3*] Type II (noninsulin-dependent) diabetes mellitus (adult onset) is related to obesity and genetic factors. Most type II patients are 15% above their ideal weight, and there is a 90%–100% concordance rate for type II diabetes mellitus in identical twins. Epinephrine, which is elevated during stress, cortisone, and thiazide diuretics are diabetogenic; if these are reduced or stopped, insulin-resistance is avoided, and blood glucose levels tend to become normal. Caloric restriction, exercise, and weight reduction also are useful in reducing blood glucose. Prednisolone, a glucocorticord, can induce steroid diabetes.

260. The answer is D. (*Pediatrics Chapter 9 III A; Surgery Chapter 33 V C 1; VI A 3*) The 1-month-old infant with a history of vomiting and constipation is most likely to have pyloric stenosis, which affects approximately 1 out of every 500 infants (boys more commonly than girls). Projectile, nonbilious vomiting is the cardinal feature, and all patients with pyloric stenosis present with it. Constipation and weight loss may also be presenting complaints. The diagnosis is made on the basis of the history and palpation of a firm, nontender mass in the right hypochondrium or epigastrium. The therapy of choice is pyloromyotomy. Acute cholecystitis is usually seen in adults and is more common in women. Volvulus neonatorum and duodenal atresia are usually associated with bile-stained vomiting. Acholuric jaundice is a hereditary condition that is associated with hemolytic anemia and jaundice; the urine does not contain bile as the hyperbilirubinemia is due to unconjugated bilirubin. This condition does not usually present with vomiting unless it is complicated by cholelithiasis, but this usually presents later in life.

261. The answer is B. (*Immunology Chapter 10 V G*) Myasthenia gravis is a chronic autoimmune disease due to neuromuscular dysfunction as a result of depletion of acetylcholine receptors at the myoneural junction. Approximately 80%–90% of patients have antibodies against the acetylcholine receptor. Signs and symptoms of this disease include muscle weakness and fatigability, affecting primarily ocular, pharyngeal, facial, skeletal, and laryngeal muscles. An enlarged thymus is seen in 60%–80% of patients.

262. The answer is D. (*Medicine Chapter 6 Part II: III B; Pathology Chapter 15 VI B 1; Surgery Chapter 7 XI D 2*) Hypokalemia is defined as serum potassium levels that are less than 3.5 mEq/L. Hypokalemia may result from an inadequate dietary intake, diarrhea, vomiting, and diuretic therapy without potassium supplementation. It is also associated with many disease states, including chronic diarrhea, villous adenoma, primary hyperaldosteronism, and Cushing's syndrome. Hyperparathyroidism is not associated with hypokalemia.

263. The answer is C. (*See Appendix for references*) The x-rays that accompany the question show air bronchograms and consolidation in the region of the right middle lobe. There is also some apical fibrosis in the right lung suggestive of old healed tuberculosis. Signs of activity of *Mycobacterium tuberculosis*, however, should be ruled out; thus, in addition to microscopy, culture of sputum and staining for acid-fast bacilli are necessary. A very high erythrocyte sedimentation rate is also suggestive of tuberculosis. Aspergillosis may cause an aspergilloma (fungus ball) and may be etiologic in the development of asthma. It is usually an opportunistic infection seen in immunocompromised patients.

264. The answer is B. (*Surgery Chapter 33 VI A; VIII B, D*) The neonate described in the question who repeatedly vomits bile-stained fluid and whose abdominal x-ray shows the classic double-bubble sign (intestinal gas in the stomach and duodenum) is most likely to have duodenal atresia—that is, failure of the second portion of the duodenum to recanalize in the embryonic stages of development. There is a high rate of other anomalies in neonates with duodenal atresia, such as trisomy 21, cardiac abnormalities, and annular pancreas. Surgery is the treatment of choice, and the results are usually good; however, many of these infants do poorly as a result of the other associated anomalies.

Meconium ileus is due to mucoviscidosis, which is associated with blockage of the pancreatic ducts and loss of tryptic digestion that results in impaction of the lower ileum with intestinal mucus and meconium. X-rays show dilated loops of bowel and a typical "mottled," ground-glass appearance of meconium. Meckel's diverticulum arises from the ileum. The blind pouch may become inflamed and may be indistinguishable from appendicitis and acute intestinal obstruction. It may also induce intussusception. However, it usually becomes symptomatic in young adult life, not in the neonatal period. Hirschsprung's disease can present with bile-stained vomit in the neonate, but radiologic examination shows air–fluid levels, a distended bowel, and often no air in the rectum.

265. The answer is D. (*See Appendix for references*) Serum alkaline phosphatase may be elevated in children (due to normal bone growth) and during pregnancy. It may also be elevated due to hepatic duct or cholangiolar obstruction and to osteoblastic bone disease, such as hyperparathyroidism, rickets, osteomalacia, Paget's disease, and neoplasia of bone (i.e., osteosarcoma or metastatic neoplasms to bone). It is also elevated when hepatotoxicity results from drugs, such as chlorpromazine and methyltestosterone. The level of serum alkaline phosphatase is decreased in hypothyroidism and in growth retardation in children.

266. The answer is D. (*Preventive Medicine and Public Health Chapter 6 I A; II A–D; Figure 6-1; Table 6-1*) Maternal mortality consists of deaths as a result of complications of pregnancy, childbirth, and the puerperium. These deaths must occur within a year of the pregnancy. Maternal mortality is higher following childbearing than it is from legal abortion, sterilization, and temporary methods of contraception combined. Analysis of United States statistics reveals the following: (1) Maternal mortality rates by age reveal somewhat higher mortality rates for younger and older women worldwide and for older women in the United States; (2) maternal mortality rates by race reveal consistently lower rates for white women than for black women and women of other races; and (3) hypertensive diseases of pregnancy, embolism, hemorrhage, infection, *and* ectopic pregnancy are major causes of maternal mortality.

267. The answer is D. (*Pathology Chapter 15 III B 2; see also Appendix for references*) The patient in the photograph that accompanies the question has a pubertal goiter due to the physiologic elevation of thyroid-stimulating hormone (TSH) as a result of iodine deficiency or stress, and thus it is remediable. She should be advised that surgery is contraindicated and to take iodized salt to optimize T_4 synthesis, which will in turn reduce TSH secretion and follicular stimulation. Radiotherapy is not indicated, and because the patient is euthyroid, propylthiouracil is also contraindicated.

268. The answer is D. [*Psychiatry Chapter 3 IV F 2 x (4); Chapter 4 III A 1*] The 32-year-old man described in the question made a desperate attempt to stop drinking, resulting in delirium tremens (alcohol withdrawal delirium), which arises after cessation or significant reduction in alcohol use.

Although alcoholics of all ages are susceptible, it is most common in individuals between 30 and 40 years of age. It occurs in fewer than 5% of alcoholics. Symptoms include impaired attention, memory, and concentration; impulsive and unpredictable behavior; tachycardia; tremulousness; diaphoresis; nausea; weakness; and orthostatic hypotension. Vivid auditory hallucinations are also characteristic of alcoholic withdrawal syndrome.

269. The answer is E. (*See Appendix for references*) Mammography is the most effective diagnostic technique to detect nonpalpable breast cancer; in fact, it can detect cancer in the breast 2 years before it becomes palpable. It may not, however, reveal medullary type cancer, and there is an increased risk of developing cancer of the breast after exposure to radiation. This risk, however, is relatively small since less than 1 rad is administered for a bilateral, two-view mammogram. For every rad of radiation to the breast, about six new cases per million women per year may result after a 10-year latent period. It has been shown, using computerized mathematical models, that the lives saved by early breast cancer detection, using mammography, exceeds 500 per million women screened. Thus, if employed judiciously, mammography has a significant role in the early detection of breast cancer. It is also important to note that evidence of breast cancer is not diagnostic even if reported by the best radiologist. Biopsy and histologic confirmation are mandatory.

270. The answer is D. (*Pathology Chapter 19 I H 3; see also Appendix for references*) Osteogenic sarcoma is a highly malignant bone tumor that affects young men between the ages of 10 and 20 years. It is the second most common primary tumor after multiple myeloma. Ninety percent of primary osteogenic sarcomas involve the appendicular skeleton (i.e., femur, humerus, and tibia), but they can involve any bone. This tumor affects mainly the metaphyseal end of long bones. It invades the soft tissue, spreading outside the confines of normal bone and is deposited as irregular spicules of bone, radiating away from the shaft, giving a "sun ray" or "sunburst" effect radiologically (see figure below). As the tumor grows, the periosteum is elevated, and reactive bone formation takes place below the periosteum and above the tumor. Radiologically, this tumor is seen as a triangle; however, Codman's triangle is not pathognomonic.

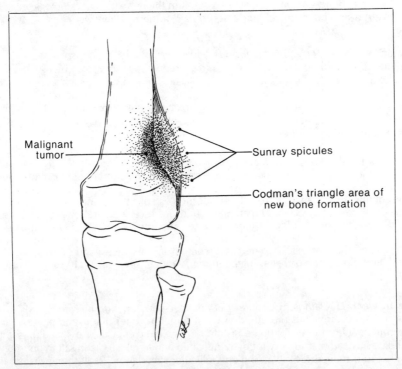

271. The answer is D. [*Pharmacology, 2nd ed, Chapter 11 III D 1 f (2); Chapter 12 VIII E; Surgery Chapter 30 II C 1, 2, F 1 c (2)–(4)*] Solar keratosis is best treated with 5-fluorouracil cream. It is a benign condition, although 10%–20% of lesions will undergo malignant change. Basal cell carcinoma (rodent ulcer) can be treated by wide excision or superficial radiotherapy. It is most common in elderly, white individuals in tropical regions. Bowen's disease is an intraepidermal squamous cell carcinoma, which can resemble a plaque of psoriasis. The course is relatively benign, but malignant change can occur. It is best to excise this lesion widely if possible. Tinea versicolor is a fungal infection of the skin, which is a relatively harmless condition, but pale macules on the skin can be embarrassing and difficult to treat. Ketoconazole (200 mg daily for 2–4 weeks) yields a 90% success rate, but hepatotoxicity may result. Pityriasis rosea is a self-limited eruption possibly of viral etiology.

272 and 273. The answers are: 272-B, 273-C. (*Pediatrics Chapter 9 VII A 5*) The 9-month-old infant described in the question who presents with colicky abdominal pain and red "currant jelly" stools is suffering from intussusception, that is, invagination of part of the intestine into another part. Patients classically present with colicky pain, vomiting, lethargy, red "currant jelly" stools, and a palpable tubular mass. Intussusception is one of the most common causes of intestinal obstruction in children up to 2 years of age. A barium enema will show a coiled-spring appearance to the bowel, which is diagnostic. Hydrostatic reduction by a careful barium enema performed by an experienced radiologist is successful in about 75% of cases.

274. The answer is E. (*See Appendix for references*) Rupture of the uterus is one of the most serious obstetric accidents, accounting for 5% of maternal deaths. Rupture may occur either before labor or during labor as a result of rupture of a previous cesarean section scar or previous operative scar, trauma to the uterus, and spontaneous rupture of the uterus. Spontaneous rupture of the uterus is most likely to occur in multiparous women, women with cephalopelvic disproportion, and in women in the older age groups. Hypotonic uterine inertia is unlikely to cause uterine rupture.

275. The answer is D. [*Preventive Medicine and Public Health Chapter 12 IV C 1 a (3); Psychiatry Chapter 3 IV F 2 y (2) (g)*] Asbestos, which is used as insulation and in roofing materials and automotive parts, has been implicated as a causative factor in the following diseases: interstitial pulmonary fibrosis; pleural plaques and effusion; lung, laryngeal, and gastrointestinal cancer; and mesothelioma. Nasal septal ulceration may occur as a complication of cocaine abuse by inhalation (snorting).

276. The answer is C. (*Anatomy Chapter 32 III A 7; Immunology Chapter 10 V G; Pediatrics Chapter 16 IX B 6 b; XI F 2*) Bell's palsy is probably a postinfectious seventh cranial nerve neuropathy due to inflammation in the facial canal, resulting in paralysis of the muscles of expression. Ipsilateral expressionless drooping of the face and the ipsilateral paralysis of orbicularis oculi and oris result in the inability to close the eyelids and to smile, respectively. A lesion of the eighth cranial nerve results in deafness. Paralysis agitans (parkinsonism) is due to a lesion in the substantia nigra and is associated with "pill-rolling" tremor and hypokinesia. Myasthenia gravis may present with droopy eyelids, muscular weakness, and fatigability; it is due to faulty neuromuscular transmission. Huntington's chorea is due to abnormalities in the basal ganglia and is associated with choreoathetosis, dystonia, and rigidity.

277. The answer is E. [*Pathology Chapter 14 VIII A 1, 2; Surgery Chapter 23 III A 3 h (2), B 3 b*] The American Cancer Society recommends that the first or baseline mammogram should be done by age 35–40 years (or earlier, if a personal or family history of breast cancer is present). Also, because there is an increased risk of breast cancer in women with uterine cancer, they should be evaluated regularly with a mammogram. Also, patients with a breast cyst should have a mammogram or ultrasound before aspiration or biopsy. Mammography is a valuable tool in the early detection of breast cancer, but it must be used judiciously. There is no current evidence that exogenous estrogens per se are causative agents in breast cancer; however, estrogens are known to support the growth of a preexisting breast neoplasm.

278. The answer is C. [*Pharmacology, 2nd ed, Chapter 3 II A 6 e; V B 6 c (1); Chapter 4 III A 2 b (5); Chapter 10 II C 2 h; Chapter 12 IX A 7 e*] Phenobarbital decreases serum bilirubin levels and has been used in neonates to prevent physiologic jaundice and to treat hyperbilirubinemia. It also is used to reduce serum bilirubin levels in older children and adults with familial nonhemolytic, nonobstructive jaundice. It is the ability of barbiturates to stimulate hepatic glucuronyl transferase that underlies its use in the treatment of hyperbilirubinemia and kernicterus in the newborn.

Halothane, a fluorinated gas, is the most widely used of the volatile anesthetic agents. There is evidence that it may cause severe postoperative liver dysfunction, including jaundice and death, when repeated exposure occurs over a 4- to 6-week period. This complication, which is rare, may be caused by reduced metabolites of halothane. Other hepatotoxic drugs include chlorpromazine, an antipsychotic; isoniazid, an antituberculosis drug; and oral contraceptives.

92

279. The answer is D. (*Medicine Chapter 5 VII A; Surgery Chapter 7 XVII; Chapter 9 II F; Chapter 10 II*) The 24-year-old student described in the question who presents with severe abdominal pain and nausea is most likely suffering from acute pancreatitis. Most cases (70%) of acute pancreatitis are due either to gallstones or to the abuse of alcohol. The clinical presentation involves severe, steady abdominal pain in the periumbilical region that may radiate to the back, nausea, vomiting, and abdominal tenderness. Alcohol stimulates gastrin release, which results in gastric hyperacidity, which results in increased pancreatic secretion and spasm of the sphincter of Oddi. Mesenteric adenitis is usually associated with an upper respiratory tract infection, and the pain does not usually radiate to the back. Acute diverticulitis is usually seen in older patients with a history of chronic constipation and pain in the left lower quadrant of the abdomen. In appendicitis, the pain begins in the epigastrium and moves to the umbilical region; over a period of 1–12 hr, appendiceal pain localizes in the right iliac fossa. Pain that radiates directly to the back from the epigastrium is usually characteristic of pancreatitis or perforated peptic ulcer, although other studies, such as serum amylase or serum calcium, are necessary to arrive at a definitive diagnosis. Acute cholecystitis is seen most frequently in women between 30–80 years of age. Pain is usually in the epigastrium and right upper quadrant and radiates into the infrascapular region.

280. The answer is A. (*Pathology Chapter 19 I B 1 b, G 1 a–c*) Paget's disease of the bone (osteitis deformans) is characterized by excessive bone destruction and repair (turnover), resulting in deformities because the repair is disorganized. The high turnover is characterized by the presence of numerous osteoclasts and osteoblasts, an increased calcification rate, and accumulation of woven bones. The head may become large, and headaches and bone pain may occur. Expansion of bone may result in VIII nerve compression and thus cause nerve deafness. Serum calcium and phosphate levels are normal, and the alkaline phosphatase is elevated. The long bones may be involved, resulting in bowing of the legs. There is usually increased vascularity of the bones, which act as multiple atrioventricular fistulas, resulting in high output cardiac failure. Paget's disease affects 3%–4% of the population over 40 years of age, particularly men. Blue discoloration of sclerae is not a feature of Paget's disease. It is seen in osteogenesis imperfecta tarda, which is an autosomal dominant trait manifested by a predisposition toward multiple bone fractures.

281 and 282. The answers are: 281-E, 282-A. (*Microbiology Chapter 21 III D; Pediatrics Chapter 8 V H 5 a; Chapter 14 I C 2 a; Surgery Chapter 11 V I 4*) Fever, sore throat, lymphadenopathy, and a positive Paul-Bunnell test confirm the diagnosis of infectious mononucleosis, an acute infection caused by the Epstein-Barr virus (EBV). The diagnosis of infectious mononucleosis is made on the basis of the clinical presentation, characteristic blood abnormalities, heterophil agglutination tests (Paul-Bunnell test), and EBV antibody titers.

Infectious mononucleosis presents in three clinical stages: (1) a nonspecific prodromal stage that lasts 3–6 days; (2) the midstage that lasts approximately 4–20 days, during which the full-blown syndrome presents itself; and (3) convalescence. Splenomegaly occurs in approximately 50% of patients, and this predisposes to rupture of the spleen, following even minor trauma. Thus, the abdomen must be examined with care.

An urgent laparotomy is indicated because the patient has gone into shock, which indicates a massive internal hemorrhage, due to possible rupture of the spleen.

283. The answer is E. (*Medicine Chapter 3 I A 1 c; Chapter 5 I B 2 c; Pediatrics Chapter 13 III C 2 c*) Iron deficiency anemia is the only anemia in which hemosiderin is absent in bone marrow. It may present with soft, thin, and brittle nails (koilonychia); fatigue; weakness; glossitis; and dysphagia, a condition known as Plummer-Vinson (Paterson-Kelly) syndrome. A positive diagnosis is made from an absence of marrow iron on bone marrow examination, abnormally low levels of ferritin, and low serum iron in association with an elevated total iron-binding capacity.

284. The answer is B. (*Medicine Chapter 3 V D 1 a; Pathology Chapter 17 III B 1; Pediatrics Chapter 13 VI F*) Classic hemophilia (hemophilia A) is associated with a normal bleeding time (except after aspirin ingestion) and also normal capillary fragility, prothrombin time, fibrinogen content, and platelet count. The coagulation time may range from 30 min to several hours. Partial thromboplastin time is markedly prolonged. Antihemophilic factor is virtually absent from the plasma, and, therefore, thromboplastin cannot be formed. Hemophilia A is transmitted as a classic X-linked recessive trait by clinically unaffected women carriers to men offspring. Women carriers may be identified by low or low-normal levels of factor VIII:C(pro) with normal levels of factor VIII:R(ag). About 85% of congenital bleeders have hemophilia A; in one-third of these cases, the occurrence is sporadic with no history in the family of a bleeding disorder. Hemophilia A may present with recurrent hemarthroses and hematomas, often resulting after minor injury. These may be treated with fresh, frozen plasma.

285. The answer is C. (*Medicine Chapter 9 III A, B*) Sarcoidosis may cause hypercalcemia because the granulomatous tissue produces 1,25-dihydroxyvitamin D_3. Hypercalcemia is also caused by hyperparathyroidism, acute immobilization, vitamin D intoxication, milk alkali syndrome, and acute adrenal insufficiency. It may also be associated with neoplastic conditions, such as bronchogenic carcinoma, breast carcinoma, multiple myeloma, adrenal carcinoma, and prostatic carcinoma. Reduced total and ionized calcium, that is, true hypocalcemia, may be due to vitamin D deficiency, acute pancreatitis, magnesium deficiency, hyperphosphatemia, hypoparathyroidism, pseudohypoparathyroidism, and renal tubular acidosis. Hypoalbuminemia is the most common cause of reduced total serum calcium concentration, although the ionized calcium level is normal, and no treatment is indicated.

286. The answer is B. (*Psychiatry Chapter 3 IV D 3 a; see also Appendix for references*) Alzheimer's disease is a primary degenerative dementia that may occur at any age but usually manifests between the ages of 50 and 60 years. It usually develops insidiously and may present with amnesia and dementia accompanied by delirium, delusions, or depression; however, no symptom complex is particularly characteristic. The presence of a Kayser-Fleischer ring is not pathognomonic of Alzheimer's disease but is pathognomonic of Wilson's disease, an autosomal recessive metabolic disorder of copper metabolism, resulting in hepatolenticular degeneration.

287. The answer is E. (*Microbiology Chapter 24 III D 2; Chapter 25 I C; see also Appendix for references*) Sleeping sickness, or African trypanosomiasis, is caused by trypanosomes of the *Trypanosoma* species. This protozoa is ingested by the tsetse fly and then transmitted to humans and animals by the bite of the fly. Clinical characteristics of sleeping sickness include parasitemia, vasculitis, lymphadenopathy, and panencephalitis. Parasitemia is accompanied by fever, tachycardia, splenomegaly, skin rash, and headache; a chancre often appears at the site of inoculation. Diagnosis is made by microscopically examining lymph node aspirates, blood, or cerebrospinal fluid for trypanosomes. Serologic tests for syphilis may be falsely positive in patients with African trypanosomiasis. Periorbital edema, muscle tenderness, and barrel-shaped eggs in stools are characteristic of trichuriasis infection.

288. The answer is C. (*Obstetrics and Gynecology Chapter 21 I A, B; Chapter 22 I A–C*) The menstrual cycle can be divided into three phases. Phase 1, the follicular phase, is a relatively infertile phase; it extends from the first day of menstrual bleeding to the beginning of the development of the egg follicle. This phase varies in length from cycle to cycle. Phase 2, the fertile phase, extends from the beginning of follicular development until 48 hours after ovulation. Since spermatozoa can fertilize the ovum for up to 5 days in the cervical mucus, the fertile phase lasts 6–8 days a cycle. The luteal phase extends from ovulation to the onset of menstruation, and the absolutely infertile phase extends from 48 hours after ovulation to the onset of menstruation. The luteal phase is of a fairly constant duration, lasting 10–16 days, but usually only 14. Thus, the woman in the question whose menstrual cycles are 34 days long should be told that she is most likely to ovulate on day 20 of her cycle. To be definite about the fertile period, it is important to consider the fact that ovulation may take place on day 24, and allowing another 48 hours after ovulation, it would be safe after day 26. Although the fertile phase extends from the beginning of follicular development and lasts 6 to 8 days a cycle, this is variable. Thus, ovulation could take place at the other extreme, that is, on day 18. The fertile period then would be between days 18 and 26. To be extra careful, especially because the follicular phase is less consistent than the luteal phase, one could say that the fertile period in this woman would be day 16 to day 26, during which time she should abstain from sex.

289. The answer is A. (*Obstetrics and Gynecology Chapter 29 I; II D; see also Appendix for references*) An ectopic pregnancy is any pregnancy that implants anyplace besides the endometrial lining of the uterine cavity, such as the oviduct, cervix, fallopian tubes, ovary, or abdomen. Most ectopic pregnancies, however, are tubal pregnancies (95%). Ectopic pregnancy is most common among nonwhite populations, implicating previous pelvic inflammatory disease as a causative factor. A high percentage of pregnancies conceived with an intrauterine device (IUD) in place are ectopic; however, these appear to be related to the efficiency of the device in preventing uterine pregnancies rather than from a particular relationship of the IUD to ectopic pregnancy. Common presenting signs and symptoms include amenorrhea followed by abnormal uterine bleeding, signs and symptoms of pregnancy, unilateral pelvic pain, fainting, and exquisite tenderness on vaginal examination. Cullen's sign, a bluish discoloration of the umbilicus that indicates intraperitoneal hemorrhage, is rare and may only be seen in women with an umbilical hernia or in women who are thin.

290. The answer is A. (*Medicine Chapter 3 V; Table 3-1*) Prothrombin time (PT) measures mainly the "extrinsic system" of the coagulation cascades. A prolonged PT indicates a deficiency of one or more extrinsic system factors or the presence of an inhibitor. PT is prolonged by warfarin. The coagulation cascade of both the extrinsic and intrinsic pathways is depicted below.

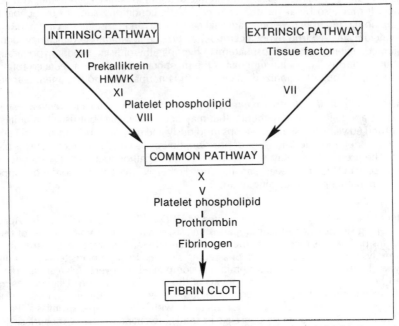

Adapted from Wintrobe MM, et al: *Clinical Hematology*, 8th ed. Philadelphia, Lea and Febiger, 1981, p 418.

291. The answer is D. (*Medicine Chapter 9 V B 2 a–g, 3 b*) Cushing's syndrome may be due to hyperplasia or tumor, which results in adrenocortical hyperfunction. Classically, the patient may present with centripetal obesity, easy bruising, psychosis, hirsutism, and purple striae. There is muscle wasting and weakness (not hypertrophy) due to the catabolic effect of excessive cortisol on muscle protein. The patient may have hypertension, glycosuria, and osteoporosis. The serum potassium and chloride are low, and the 17-hydroxycorticosteroids are elevated. Administration of exogenous dexamethasone does not suppress secretion of cortisol. Red and white cell counts may be elevated with a lymphocytopenia and low total eosinophil count. Cushing's syndrome may also be associated with psychotic disturbances, especially depression. The hallmark of Cushing's syndrome is hypercortisolism, which can be caused by a neoplasm of the pituitary (Cushing's disease), adrenal cortex, or an ectopic site, such as the lung (e.g., oat cell, or bronchogenic, carcinoma).

292. The answer is E. [*Obstetrics and Gynecology Chapter 36 III A, B; Pathology Chapter 14 VIII A 1, 2; Surgery Chapter 23 III A 3 d, h (2)*] Currently, there is no evidence that links breast cancer to exogenous estrogens; however, there may be an association with endometrial cancer, which *is* linked to estrogen (unopposed by progesterone) use. Estrogens can be administered to women with metastatic breast carcinoma who are more than 5 years *past* menopause, and they may induce remissions of variable length in some patients. Risk factors for breast cancer include a positive family history for breast cancer, history of chronic cystic mastitis, previous breast cancer, high socioeconomic status, nulliparity, and first full-term pregnancy after 35 years of age.

293. The answer is E. (*See Appendix for references*) Herpes simplex viruses (HSV-1 and HSV-2) are DNA viruses that are found worldwide. It is believed that HSV-1 virus lies dormant in the trigeminal ganglion after the primary infection and flares up when an individual's resistance is low. Although HSV-2 is usually responsible for genital herpes, HSV-1 can cause genital herpes as well. However, a painful balanitis is usually caused by a HSV-2 infection. HSV-1 is most often contracted from family members during childhood. Some studies have reported 40%–90% of individuals have HSV-1 antibodies. HSV-2 antibodies are not usually evident until puberty and then only in sexually active adolescents. The incubation period for HSV-1 infection is most often 3–7 days but can be as long as 20 days.

294. The answer is E. (*Pediatrics Chapter 1 VI D 1; see also Appendix for references*) The first words that an infant speaks are nouns, most commonly "dada" and "mama," at about 10 months of age, although not necessarily to indicate a parent; such specific references occur at about 12 to 15 months of age. By 18 months, toddlers will use several words, including verbs, and they are able to identify body parts when named. By 2 years of age, adjectives and pronouns are used, and two or more words are combined into short sentences. If by the age of 2 years the child does not speak, the child should be evaluated for a congenital hearing defect or other neuromuscular defect, or even for a psychosocial problem, such as emotional deprivation. By 3 years of age, verbalizations reach an average of 200 words.

295. The answer is E. [*Obstetrics and Gynecology Chapter 15 I B 4, 5; Pathology Chapter 16 II D 2 b (1); Preventive Medicine and Public Health Chapter 10 IV B; see also Appendix for references*] Neonates with congenital toxoplasmosis present with microcephaly or hydrocephaly, seizures, convulsions, mental retardation, hepatosplenomegaly, cerebral calcification, and chorioretinitis, resulting in blindness. The mother is often asymptomatic, but the fetus is almost always infected. Manifestations of early congenital syphilis include bullous eruptions on the palms and soles in the neonate.

296. The answer is A. (*Surgery Chapter 12 II A; Chapter 18 III E; Chapter 25 XII A 3 a*) The man described in the question who presents with a mass on the left side of the neck is most likely to have a carotid body tumor. Carotid body tumors (paragangliomas, also known as potato tumors) are usually benign, painless masses that grow very slowly. While paragangliomas are rarely malignant (2%–6%), local invasion can be extensive. The mass may or may not have a bruit, and large tumors can result in dysphagia, obstruction of the airway, and cranial nerve palsies. Thyroglossal cysts usually present as midline masses between the hyoid bone and the thyroid isthmus that move upward when the patient is asked to put out the tongue; they are most often seen in children. Cystic hygromas are brilliantly translucent neck tumors that occur during the first year of life. Carotid artery aneurysm will normally present as a pulsatile swelling with a thrill that can be palpated; auscultation would reveal a bruit due to turbulence in blood flow caused by aneurysmal dilation. Tuberculous lymph nodes are usually tender and firm and adhere to one another; breakdown of the overlying skin sometimes results in stubborn draining sinuses, which heal with scarring.

297. The answer is A. (*See Appendix for references*) Herpes simplex virus type 2 (HSV-2) is usually acquired in puberty after the initiation of sexual activity. (HSV-1 is usually acquired during childhood.) The primary infection, just as with HSV-1, is usually the most severe episode. It is accompanied by pain, itching, dysuria, inguinal adenopathy, lesions on the external genitalia, fever, headache, myalgia, and vaginal and urethral discharge. The primary infection usually lasts longer and has a higher rate of complications than subsequent infections. There is no known vaccine for primary prevention although acyclovir may shorten the duration of the lesions and other symptoms. Latent infections are triggered by menstruation, anxiety, or illness. There appears to be some cross-immunity between HSV-1 and HSV-2 that confers partial protection with the heterologous antigenic virus.

298. The answer is B. [*Anatomy Chapter 22 VI D 1 e (2), 2 b (2); Obstetrics and Gynecology Chapter 32 III A, E; see also Appendix for references*] Fertilization normally occurs in the outer one-third of the fallopian tube. The ovum, surrounded by the zona pellucida, is bombarded by many spermatozoa, only one of which actually penetrates the ovum. After 3 to 3½ days, the fertilized ovum sheds the zona pellucida and reaches the uterus for nidation (implantation).

299–301. The answers are: 299-E, 300-D, 301-D. (*Medicine Chapter 2 XIV A; see also Appendix for references*) The x-rays that accompany the question show hilar lymphadenopathy. The history indicates an anergy to tuberculin and negative sputum examination for acid-fast bacilli. Sarcoidosis is a noncaseating chronic granulomatous, multiorgan disease that can cause paratracheal and hilar lymphadenopathy. It is associated with a complete anergy to tuberculin (due to impaired cellular immunity) and elevated serum calcium levels that are lowered by the administration of steroids. (Hyperkalemia causes peaked narrow T waves, a widening QRS complex, a shortened QT interval, and prominent U waves). Hypercalcemia can cause various cardiac abnormalities and classically causes shortened QT intervals on electrocardiogram. Aspergillosis, which is usually seen in immunocompromised patients, presents as an aspergilloma and asthma. Carcinoma of the bronchus may cause hilar lymphadenopathy, but there is usually pathology evident, and no malignant cells have been reported on microscopy. Also, carcinoma of the bronchus is usually seen in older patients with a history of smoking.

302. The answer is C. (*See Appendix for references*) The causative organism for the lesion that is discharging pus is likely to be *Actinomyces israelii*, an anaerobic bacteria that can cause cervicofacial abscesses. These abscesses eventually rupture to form sinus tracts that exude characteristic sulfur granules in the pus. The drug of first choice is penicillin G; tetracycline and chloramphenicol may also be effective. However, definitive cure may also necessitate drainage or excision of the lesion.

303. The answer is D. [*Pediatrics Chapter 6 III E 4 a (4); Preventive Medicine and Public Health Chapter 10 IV A 3*] Down's syndrome occurs as a result of an extra chromosome 21 (trisomy 21) because of (1) a failure in chromosomal pairing of one of the parental germ cells, (2) a translocation when the long arm of chromosome 21 becomes attached to another chromosome (13, 18, or another 21), and (3) trisomy mosaic 21 in which only some cells are trisomic and the rest are normal. Common clinical features include mental retardation (most patients have IQs below 50); flat facial profile; short, upslanting palpebral fissures; Brushfield's spots; a flat nasal bridge with epicanthal folds; a small mouth with protruding tongue; a small, retroplaced chin; and short ears with abnormal ear lobes that are usually downfolded. The functional characteristics of Down's syndrome include hyperflexible joints and hypotonic muscle. Other clinical features include microcephaly, flat occiput (bradycephaly), excess posterior neck skin, short stature, short sternum, small genitalia, short hands and fingers marked by incurved fifth fingers with a hypoplastic middle phalanx, single (simian) palmar creases, and a gap between the first and the second toes. The "setting sun" sign is usually due to hydrocephalus.

304 and 305. The answers are: 304-D, 305-C. (*Medicine Chapter 8 VI C 1–3; see also Appendix for references*) The clinical presentation of an emaciated man who complains of night sweats, weight loss, and lethargy characterizes a debilitating condition. The distended abdomen implies ascites, which would cause a "fluid thrill" on physical examination. Because there are few options available, it would be wise to make a provisional diagnosis of tuberculosis and treat the patient with ethambutol, isoniazid, and streptomycin and monitor the patient's progress (i.e., chart daily weight and temperature and repeat the erythrocyte sedimentation rate every 7 days). Ethambutol can cause retrobulbar neuritis with reduced visual acuity—the earliest manifestation being a decreased ability to perceive the color green. This may be bilateral or unilateral; therefore, each eye should be checked separately. This complication resolves after withdrawal from the drug. Streptomycin is potentially ototoxic. Isoniazid may cause peripheral neuropathy, convulsions, psychosis, ataxia, dizziness, and optic neuritis. These side effects occur infrequently and are dose-related. The neuropathy may be prevented by administering pyridoxine.

306. The answer is A. (*See Appendix for references*) Modern mammography is a very effective diagnostic tool for the early diagnosis of a nonpalpable breast cancer. However, there is an increased risk of developing breast cancer after exposure to radiation. About 6 new cases of breast cancer per million women per year for every rad of radiation may result after a 10-year latent period. However, it has been shown from computerized mathematical models that the lives saved by early breast cancer detection using mammography exceeded 500 per million women screened. This differential is further improved with improved image resolution and decreased radiation exposure. Thus, the average breast x-ray dose should not exceed 1 rad for a two-view bilateral mammogram.

307. The answer is A. (*Preventive Medicine and Public Health Chapter 10 IV A 1 b*) Maple syrup urine disease is associated with severe neurologic damage and mental retardation, occurring in the early neonatal period and usually leading to an early death. The biochemical defect interferes with decarboxylation of the branched-chain amino acids (i.e., leucine, isoleucine, and valine), which accumulate in the blood, causing aminoaciduria. The urine has a characteristic odor (maple syrup) from the derivatives of the keto acids.

308. The answer is B. [*Medicine Chapter 6 Part II III B 2 b (1), (2), C 2 a (2); see also Appendix for references*] Hyperkalemia is characterized by a serum potassium concentration greater than 5.5 mEq/L. Blood, especially that stored for 10 days or more, has a high potassium ion content in plasma (i.e., as much as 30 mEq/L), which may result in hyperkalemia after administration. Thiazide diuretics, amphotericin B, carbenicillin, and excessive licorice consumption may be associated with hypokalemia.

309. The answer is E. (*Obstetrics and Gynecology Chapter 22 III E; Chapter 29 II D; III A, B*) The most likely diagnosis for the woman described in the question with acute pain and uterine bleeding is an ectopic pregnancy. There is a greater chance that a pregnancy will be ectopic if an intrauterine device (IUD) is in place than if no IUD is used, possibly because the IUD is so effective in preventing a uterine pregnancy. The most common presenting complaint of an ectopic pregnancy is abnormal uterine bleeding, which is often interpreted by the patient as a delayed period, particularly as bleeding often occurs 7–14 days after a missed menstrual period. Bleeding is often accompanied by unilateral pelvic pain that can be either sharp or dull. The signs and symptoms of acute appendicitis and Meckel's diverticulitis cannot be distinguished by clinical examination except by exploration. Acute salpingitis may be associated with vaginal discharge, which may be purulent and offensive. Crohn's disease may present like appendicitis, but there may be associated findings, such as perianal fistulas. Ectopic pregnancy would be difficult to distinguish from appendicitis, but the patient is usually shocked and in great danger due to the internal hemorrhage.

310. The answer is E. (*Pediatrics Chapter 5 V A 2 f*) Hyaline membrane disease (neonatal respiratory distress syndrome) is a respiratory disorder seen in premature infants and infants born to diabetic mothers, which is characterized by a deficiency of surfactant that makes the immature lungs poorly compliant. Conventional therapy consists of the administration of oxygen and supportive care; however, it is important to note that mechanical ventilation that raises oxygen levels over 40% may cause fibroplasia, resulting in partial or total blindness.

311. The answer is A. (*Pediatrics Chapter 8 VII E; X B*) Chickenpox is a contagious varicella zoster infection that affects primarily children under 10 years of age. Patients present with fever, malaise, anorexia, and pruritic vesicular eruptions. These eruptions occur in "crops" so that the lesions are often in several different stages at the same time. Although the diagnosis can be made from the clinical presentation, the Tzanck test performed on scrapings from the base of a vesicle, which shows multinucleated giant cells with intranuclear inclusions, is diagnostic. Herpes zoster represents a reactivation of the varicella infection and occurs mainly in adults; it usually affects the dermatome unilaterally. Scabies is caused by a round mite, which produces an intensely itchy rash that is worse at night; it affects mainly flexures, finger webs, and the space between the buttocks.

312. The answer is C. (*Medicine Chapter 3 V; Table 3-1; Figure 3-1*) Partial thromboplastin time (PTT) measures mainly the "intrinsic pathway" of the coagulation cascade. The PTT depends on glass activation of factor XII. All coagulation factors except platelet factor III, factor VII, and factor XIII are measured by PTT. Any break in the cardiovascular system is sealed off by the coagulation process, which can be summarized as follows:

$$\text{Prothrombin} + \text{calcium ion } (Ca^{2+}) + \text{thromboplastin} = \text{thrombin}$$
$$\text{Fibrinogen} + \text{thrombin} = \text{fibrin (which polymerizes to form a clot)}$$

Any substance that binds Ca^{2+} will prevent clotting (e.g., oxalate or citrate).

313. The answer is B. (*See Appendix for references*) Acanthosis nigricans is a symmetrical hyperpigmented, hyperkeratotic change in the epidermis of intertriginous areas (e.g., axillae, anogenital region, umbilicus, and breast). It is usually associated with internal neoplasms, such as gastric adenocarcinomas, especially in elderly individuals. It may also be associated with endocrine disorders, such as diabetes mellitus, Addison's disease, Stein-Leventhal syndrome, and acromegaly. Because this skin disorder is a significant marker for malignancy, it is important to try to locate a neoplasm as a possible etiologic factor and to institute definitive treatment. Melasma gravidarum, also referred to as chloasma of pregnancy, is associated with areas of patchy hyperpigmentation of the face.

314. The answer is A. (*Preventive Medicine and Public Health Chapter 5 IV A 1, 2, 4; Table 5-1; Surgery Chapter 23 III A 1*) Breast cancer is one of the most common cancers affecting women—that is, 9% of all women by the age of 70 will have breast cancer. It should be noted, however, that the incidence of lung cancer is increasing faster among American women than among American men. Vaginal cancer is seen in women between the ages of 60 and 70 years and accounts for 1%–2% of all gynecologic malignancies. Cancer of the cervix is more common than cancer of the uterus, but less common than breast cancer. The incidence of cervical cancer has been decreasing during the last decade. Ovarian cancer represents 4% of all invasive cancers occurring in women, and in 1981, it was the fourth leading cause of death among women with cancer.

315. The answer is B. (*Obstetrics and Gynecology Chapter 15 II D 4; Table 15-2; Preventive Medicine and Public Health Chapter 10 IV B 2 b*) The fetal alcohol syndrome is associated with maternal alcohol abuse during pregnancy. As little as 1 oz or more per day during the *first* trimester may result in some if not all of the features of prenatal alcohol exposure. Alcohol is fetotoxic because the fetal liver is immature and cannot metabolize alcohol. At birth the child manifests a typical facies, including flattened facial features, a short palpebral fissure, a long philtrum, and a smooth, thin upper lip. In addition, these children may exhibit microcephaly, developmental delay, and mental retardation. Deafness is not a feature of the fetal alcohol syndrome.

316. The answer is A. (*See Appendix for references*) Pityriasis rosea is a skin eruption of unknown etiology, but it may be caused by a picornavirus. It usually affects young adults in the spring or fall, causing oval, fawn-colored macules approximately 0.5 cm in diameter. These eruptions follow the cleavage lines of the trunk, causing a characteristic "Christmas tree" pattern. This condition is usually preceded by a slightly larger eruption known as the "herald patch" about 1–2 weeks before the florid eruption. These eruptions may be mistaken for secondary syphilis; however, the fluorescent treponemal antibody absorption test is negative. There is complete resolution in about 8 weeks without treatment.

317. The answer is C (2, 4). (*See Appendix for references*) Melasma is a hyperpigmentation that occurs most frequently to areas exposed to the sun, such as the cheeks, temples, and forehead. Although the etiology of melasma is unknown, it is most often associated with pregnancy ("the mask of pregnancy"), ovarian carcinoma, or ingestion of oral contraceptives. Lesions range in color from medium to dark brown, becoming darker with exposure to sunlight. Syphilis does not cause melasma, but it can cause leukoderma, a localized loss of melanin pigmentation. Gold and arsenic may also result in leukoderma.

318. The answer is A (1, 2, 3). (*Surgery Chapter 10 II C 5 a–c*) A patient with acute pancreatitis may present with mild abdominal discomfort to profound shock with hypotension and hypoxemia. Most commonly patients complain of nausea, vomiting, and epigastric pain that radiates to the back. Poor prognostic indicators include: age over 55 years, white blood cell count over 16,000/mm^3, anion base deficit over 4 mEq/L, arterial PO_2 below 60 mm Hg, serum glutamic oxaloacetic transaminase over 250 U/ml, serum calcium under 8 mg/dl, fasting blood sugar over 200 mg/dl, and serum lactic dehydrogenase over 350 U/ml. Although an elevated serum amylase is the hallmark of acute pancreatitis, the level of hyperamylasemia does not correlate with the severity of the pancreatitis, as many other clinical states can cause elevated serum amylase levels (e.g., bowel ischemia, obstruction, or perforation; liver and kidney diseases; ruptured ectopic pregnancy; and sialadenitis). Normal serum values for amylase and lactic dehydrogenase are 4–25 U/ml and 60–120 U/ml, respectively.

319. The answer is A (1, 2, 3). (*Pediatrics Chapter 6 III E 4 a; Chapter 14 I C 1 d*) Ninety-five percent of cases of Down's syndrome are due to tisomy 21—that is, three copies of chromosome 21 are present. Five percent of cases are due to translocations of chromosomes 21 or 22. Down's syndrome (trisomy 21) is the most frequent autosomal anomaly with an incidence of 1 in 200 newborns born to mothers 25 years of age and 1 in 100 newborns born to mothers 40 years old or older. Advanced maternal age (> 35 years) is responsible for 75% of cases of Down's syndrome, and advanced paternal age (> 35 years) is responsible for 25% of cases. However, it should be noted that most children with trisomy 21 continue to be born to women younger than 35 years of age because most women have their children before this age. The clinical presentation of Down's syndrome is the same regardless of the cause; physical examination alone cannot distinguish the underlying defect. Children with Down's syndrome have an incidence of leukemia that is 15 times greater than the normal population.

320. The answer is B (1, 3). (*Obstetrics and Gynecology Chapter 11 II; Chapter 15 Table 15-2*) IgG is the only immunoglobulin capable of placental transfer to the fetus because of its small size. Warfarin, which is fetotoxic, is also freely transferred across the placenta. Placental transfer of substances is dependent on many properties of the molecule being transferred, such as ionization, configuration, and size. Large, clumped immune complexes, such as IgM and IgA, will not cross the placenta.

321. The answer is E (all). [*Immunology Chapter 6 II B 2 b (4); Chapter 9 V D 1 a; Medicine Chapter 8 IV I; V K 1; Chapter 10 III H 3 a (4); V G 2 a (4); VI H 4 a, b; Pathology Chapter 17 III A 3; Pharmacology, 2nd ed, Chapter 10 I C 3 a, 4 b, 9 a; Psychiatry Chapter 3 IV F 2 r (1)*] The glucocorticoids enhance hepatic glucose output as a result of stimulating hepatic gluconeogenesis from amino acids (e.g., alanine) liberated by the proteolytic effect of glucosteroids. These effects lead to a decrease in glucose tolerance, hyperglycemia, glycosuria, and insulin-resistance. In patients with a low insulin reserve, a "steroid diabetes" can ensue. A common side effect of corticosteroid treatment in patients with rheumatoid arthritis is osteoporosis, a decrease in the matrix and mineral phases of bone, which can account for vertebral collapse. Glucocorticoids may produce an increase in potassium ion and hydrogen ion excretion with a concomitant retention of sodium ion with a resultant hypokalemic alkalosis. These agents can mask the symptoms of bacterial and fungal infections, and appropriate antibacterial therapy should be included. Reactivation of tuberculosis in patients receiving glucosteroids is well documented. The most common complication of topical glucocorticoid therapy is cutaneous yeast infection.

322. The answer is C (2, 4). (*Immunology Chapter 10 V C 1, 2*) Hashimoto's thyroiditis is a disease that affects women between 30 and 50 years of age. It is characterized by an enlarged thyroid gland (goiter) and histologically by lymphocyte and plasma cell infiltrates with varying amounts of fibrosis and no colloid. Hypothyroidism (i.e., diminished T_3 and T_4 levels and reduced radioactive iodine uptake) becomes evident as the disease progresses. Immunologic findings include antibody to thyroid microsomal antigen, which can be detected by the complement fixation and hemagglutination tests, antibody to thyroglobulin, which can be detected by various assays, and antibody to a colloid antigen.

323. The answer is A (1, 2, 3). [*Medicine Chapter 3 I A 3 a, b, 4; II C 2 b (2); Chapter 5 I B 2 c*] Raised serum iron is characteristically associated with hemochromatosis, sideroblastic anemia, and polycythemia vera. Plummer-Vinson (Paterson-Kelly) syndrome usually is seen in premenopausal women who present with dysphagia, koilonychia (spooning of nails), glossitis, and iron deficiency anemia. Response is dramatic after instituting treatment with oral iron tablets. There may also be an associated folate deficiency, especially if the woman has been on birth control pills.

324. The answer is C (2, 4). (*Medicine Chapter 10 II B 4 a, 5, 6, c*) Pseudogout is an arthritic condition that is characterized by gout-like symptoms, such as acute swelling, pain, stiffness, and erythema. The knee is most often involved. Fever and leukocytosis can also occur. It accounts for 25% of all cases of calcium pyrophosphate dihydrate deposition disease. Aspiration of synovial fluid yields rhomboid crystals that exhibit weakly positive birefringence in red-compensated, polarized light, which is diagnostic. Colchicine can only be administered orally or intravenously; it may be beneficial in the treatment of pseudogout if given early.

325. The answer is E (all). (*Psychiatry Chapter 3 III A 1 b, c, g*) A clouded state of consciousness is an essential feature of delirium, and this reduces the patient's awareness of his environment. Delirious patients have attention deficits that can proceed to mental confusion. Delirium also presents with sensory perceptual disturbances (e.g., illusions or hallucinations), which may cause emotional and behavioral disturbances. The patient may experience vivid dreams and nightmares. Disorientation and memory impairment are also frequently seen. Although the patient rarely forgets his or her identity, the patient loses the ability to keep track of time and recent events early in delirium, and as the delirium progresses, the patient becomes disoriented with respect to place and situation followed by confusion, bewilderment, and misinterpretation.

326. The answer is C (2, 4). (*See Appendix for references*) The terrible growth on the sole of the foot pictured in the photograph that accompanies the question is certainly a malignant tumor. However, basic principles of management demand that the diagnosis be confirmed before embarking on aggressive treatment. Thus, biopsy and radiologic examination are imperative. Cancer chemotherapy and amputation can only be done after the results of biopsy are known.

327. The answer is E (all). (*See Appendix for references*) Acute intermittent porphyria is an autosomal dominant disease occurring worldwide. Characteristically, it causes intermittent abdominal and neurologic manifestations with variable severity. There is no associated cutaneous sensitivity. Four exogenous factors may convert latent disease to a manifest disease: drugs, steroids, starvation, and infection. The drugs include barbiturates, sulfonamides, griseofulvin, and estrogens, which are steroids.

328. The answer is E (all). (*Obstetrics and Gynecology Chapter 10 II A*) Predisposing factors for low birth weight infants include the following: smoking (more than 10 cigarettes a day), maternal age less than 16 years or over 40 years, and low socioeconomic status, which may involve low income, low level of education, poor nutrition, high parity, and alcohol and drug abuse.

329. The answer is E (all). (*Pediatrics Chapter 10 IV F 1–5; Surgery Chapter 17 II F 1 a*) Tetralogy of Fallot is one of the most common congenital heart diseases, accounting for 10% of all congenital cardiac lesions. It consists of the following four defects: right ventricular hypertrophy, overriding aorta, ventricular septal defect, and obstruction of the right ventricular outflow (i.e., pulmonary valve stenosis). Because of these defects, a right-to-left shunt results in desaturated blood re-entering the systemic circulation, resulting in central cyanosis. The severity of the cyanosis depends on the degree of right ventricular outflow obstruction. Signs and symptoms include cyanosis, hyperpnea, dyspnea on exertion, and a systolic murmur over the sternal border. The systolic murmur, often accompanied by a thrill, is heard parasternally in the second or third intercostal space. Surgical management is indicated.

330. The answer is B (1, 3). (*Pediatrics Chapter 6 III E 5 b*) The patient in the photograph that accompanies the question has the classic features of hypogonadism due to Klinefelter's syndrome, a sex chromosome abnormality in which men have an extra X chromosome (47,XXY). It is usually diagnosed in adulthood when the patient presents with infertility and impotence. Males are usually incompletely masculinized after puberty with gynecomastia and decreased body hair. The testes do not grow, and there is reduced sperm production and hyperplasia of the Leydig's (interstitial) cells. Although patients with Klinefelter's syndrome are often taller than other family members, their arm *span* is usually greater than the height despite the development of disproportionate leg length.

331. The answer is A (1, 2, 3). (*Pathology Chapter 8 II E 1 a–c, e; Surgery Chapter 5 V A*) Carcinoma of the stomach occurs commonly in Japan, Iceland, and the Scandinavian countries, but its incidence in the United States appears to be decreasing. It usually affects men more commonly than women, and most patients are 50 years of age or older. These tumors are asymptomatic in the early stages, but eventually anorexia, dyspepsia, weight loss, anemia, and melena occur. Endoscopy, biopsy, and cytology are useful in confirming the diagnosis. The tumor spreads via the lymphatics, and bilateral ovarian metastases (Krukenberg's tumor) is common in women. Stomach cancer is often incurable because it is not diagnosed until it is too late; however, surgery in combination with chemotherapy is recommended. Radiation therapy is not effective. Carcinomatous ulcers can only be diagnosed by biopsy of the lesion and histologic examination.

332. The answer is E (all). (*Microbiology Chapter 24 III B; Pediatrics Chapter 8 X C 3 a; Pharmacology, 2nd ed, Chapter 12 XI A 1*) Metronidazole is the treatment of choice for the treatment of infections caused by *Giardia lamblia*. Alternative treatments for giardiasis include quinacrine hydrochloride (mepacrine hydrochloride) and furazolidone. The latter drug is the only liquid, which can be used for pediatric patients. Diiodohydroxyquin, used in cases of giardiasis resistant to quinacrine, and chloroquine are of therapeutic value as antiprotozoal drugs.

333. The answer is E (all). [*Medicine Chapter 3 V D 2 b (2)*] Disseminated intravascular coagulopathy is a very common acquired coagulopathy that occurs secondary to other disease processes, such as abruptio placentae, amniotic fluid embolism, thrombotic thrombocytopenic purpura, and widespread carcinomatosis. Clinical features vary, depending on the balance between intravascular coagulation and fibrinolysis and clotting factor depletion; for example, bleeding and shock may predominate if the coagulopathy dominates as in amniotic fluid embolism, but in more chronic cases, such as carcinomatosis, thrombosis and clotting may predominate. Diagnosis is usually made by detection of decreased fibrinogen and depletion of fibrin by the presence of high titers of fibrin degradation products.

334. The answer is C (2, 4). [*Medicine Chapter 7 V D 2 a (8); Chapter 8 V H 4 b; see also Appendix for references*] Oral and genital lesions may coexist in Behçet's disease and erythema multiforme. Behçet's disease is characterized by recurrent oral and genital ulcers, uveitis, seronegative arthritis, and central nervous system abnormalities. Erythema multiforme is characterized by symmetrical violaceous macules or nodules that appear as either grouped or isolated crops. Pityriasis rosea may be caused by a picornavirus, although the exact etiology is unknown. It presents with scaly, oval eruptions that follow the cleavage lines of the trunk and result in a Christmas tree pattern. Lymphogranuloma venereum does not cause coexisting ulcers of the mouth and genitals. It is, however, the commonest cause of inflammatory stricture of the anorectal region.

335. The answer is D (4). (*Medicine Chapter 3 V C 1; Pathology Chapter 17 III C 1 a*) Thrombocytopenia (i.e., less than 300,000 platelets) is characterized by minute bleeding spots, resulting in petechial hemorrhages under the skin and in all of the organs of the body. It is the most common cause of abnormal bleeding. Although the hallmark of thrombocytopenia is the presence of petechiae, if the platelet count is very low, there may be purpura and even a hemorrhagic diathesis with a prolonged bleeding time. Thrombocytopenia is an indication for bone marrow examination. If megakaryocytes are present in bone marrow, it indicates either peripheral obstruction or pooling of platelets. The absence of megakaryocytes indicates a defect in platelet production.

336. The answer is E (all). (*Psychiatry Chapter 2 VIII A 4; see also Appendix for references*) Electroconvulsive therapy (ECT) entails electrically induced seizures of about 60 sec per seizure. The death rate is 0.08% with the use of ECT; however, properly administered, ECT is associated with a very low morbidity and mortality. Thus, it is used most often with severely depressed suicidal patients. An organic brain disorder with blurring of memory is the most common complication of ECT that resolves spontaneously. Occasionally respiratory and cardiac arrest occur; thus, some clinicians use atropine prophylactically.

337. The answer is A (1, 2, 3). [*Microbiology Chapter 22 IV D, E; Pathology Chapter 16 II D 2 d (3) (b);*

see also Appendix for references] Rabies is caused by an RNA virus (*Rhabdoviridae*). The incubation period for rabies infection can range from 4 days to many years, but in more than 90% of cases, the incubation period is 20 to 90 days. Hydrophobia is pathognomonic of rabies. Although rabies is mainly an infection of animals, it is transmitted by animal bites. It produces encephalomyelitis, which is usually fatal. The primary reservoirs of rabies include skunks, squirrels, raccoons, foxes, bats, mongooses, wolves, and jackals. Although dogs and cats are the largest source of human infection, cattle are the most commonly affected domestic animals.

338. The answer is B (1, 3). (*Obstetrics and Gynecology Chapter 7 III A; Pediatrics Chapter 13 III C 2*) Iron deficiency anemia is the commonest cause of anemia in children. In infancy, deficiency results when iron stores are inadequate due to either low birth weight or a diet low in iron content, such as milk or cereals. In adolescence, rapid growth often coincides with a diet low in iron. In addition, adolescent girls begin to lose iron with the onset of menstruation. Iron deficiency anemia is not uncommon in menstruating women. In addition, the iron requirements of women who are either pregnant or lactating are considerable. For example, a pregnant woman needs 800 mg of elemental iron of which 300 mg goes to the fetus and 500 mg is used to expand the maternal red cell mass. Anemia exists with a hemoglobin of less than 10 g/dl during pregnancy and less than 12 g/dl in a menstruating woman.

339. The answer is A (1, 2, 3). (*Pediatrics Chapter 16 VIII A; see also Appendix for references*) The man in the photograph accompanying the question has neurofibromatosis (von Recklinghausen's disease), a relatively common autosomal dominant hereditary syndrome. It is characterized by café au lait macules (usually more than 5 cm but at least 1.5 cm), cutaneous neurofibromas, and multiple pigmented nodules in the iris (Lisch nodules). There may be associated neurologic manifestations, such as acoustic neuroma, optic glioma, intracranial tumors, pheochromocytoma, and skeletal abnormalities, such as bone cysts and kyphoscoliosis. The pheochromocytoma may be amenable to surgery, which may cure the secondary hypertension.

340. The answer is C (2, 4). (*See Appendix for references*) The venous pulse has three positive waves—a, c, and v—and two negative descents—x and y. The "a" wave is due to atrial contraction and becomes prominent with increased resistance to the right ventricle filling. Giant "a" waves in the jugular venous pulse may be caused by tricuspid stenosis, pulmonary hypertension, and severe cor pulmonale. In atrial fibrillation, the "a" waves disappear because there are rapid and weak contractions. The jugular venous pulse is illustrated below.

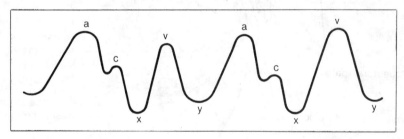

The a is an atrial contraction; c coincides with the onset of ventricular systole; v indicates a passive rise in pressure as venous return continues while the tricuspid valve is closed; y is a descent associated with a lowering of the right atrial pressure as the tricuspid valves open; and x is a descent associated with a drop in pressure in the right atrium as it relaxes with the beginning of ventricular systole, and the tricuspid valve closes.

341. The answer is E (all). (*Obstetrics and Gynecology Chapter 15 II; Table 15-2*) All of the drugs mentioned in the question are potentially teratogenic. Cyclophosphamide can cause absence of toes and flattening of the nasal bridge in the fetus. Busulfan can cause cleft palate and eye defects. Thalidomide can cause limb reduction, ear and nose abnormalities, cardiopulmonary defects, and pyloric or duodenal stenosis. Daily ingestion of pure alcohol of 1 oz or more per day during the first trimester of pregnancy can cause the fetal alcohol syndrome, which is associated with mental retardation, abnormal facies, eye and joint abnormalities, and cardiac defects in the fetus.

342. The answer is E (all). [*Pharmacology, 2nd ed, Chapter 3 IX C 1 c (3); see also Appendix for references*] Causes of hyperamylasemia include perforated peptic ulcer, mumps (sialadenitis), high intestinal obstruction, abdominal surgery, the administration of narcotics, and pancreatitis. Serum amylase is raised in 90% of patients with pancreatitis within 24 hr, but the level of increase is not useful in determining prognosis. Mumps, which is due to inflammation of the parotid glands, is associated with increased secretion of amylase. Administration of narcotics, such as morphine, may be associated with spasm of the sphincter of Oddi and obstruction of outflow of pancreatic amylase into the gastrointestinal tract with increased biliary pressure and overflow into the circulation. Perforated peptic ulceration may result in damage by acid to the pancreas and release of amylase into the circulation.

343. The answer is E (all). (*Anatomy Chapter 27 II F 6; Surgery Chapter 23 I A; see also Appendix for references*) The lymphatic drainage of the breast (see figure below) is very important, and as with any other organ, its lymphatic drainage follows the pathway of its blood supply. Therefore, it travels (1) along tributaries of the axillary vessels to the axillary lymph nodes and the supraclavicular and infraclavicular nodes and (2) along perforating branches of the internal mammary chain to the internal thoracic nodes. The breast drains principally to the axillary lymph node chain, and where axillary lymph nodes are affected by disease, approximately 48% of cases have involvement of lymph nodes along the internal mammary artery.

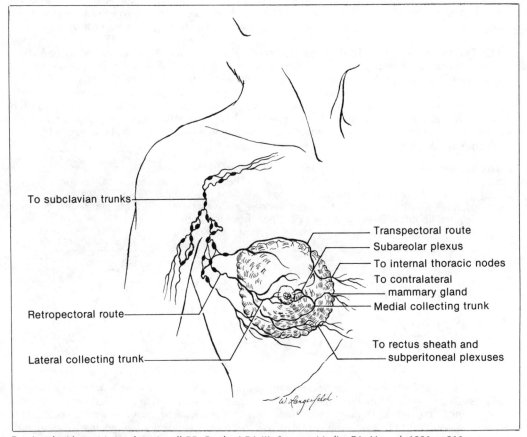

Reprinted with permission from Jarrell BE, Carabasi RA III: *Surgery*. Media, PA, Harwal, 1986, p 316.

344. The answer is E (all). (*Preventive Medicine and Public Health Chapter 11 II A; Psychiatry Chapter 4 IV A–C*) Alcohol abuse or dependence is the most serious drug problem in the United States, affecting more than 9 million Americans or 10% of the population. Three principal patterns of chronic alcohol abuse include: (1) regular daily excessive drinking; (2) regular excessive drinking on weekends only; and (3) long periods of sobriety interspersed with binges. Diagnostic clues to alcoholism include binge drinking, blackouts, inability to decrease or stop drinking, continued drinking despite the exacerbation of physical illness, drinking in the morning, apparent sobriety in the presence of an elevated alcohol level, abstinence syndromes, and solitary drinking.

345. The answer is C (2, 4). (*Pediatrics Chapter 1 IV C 8 a; V C 7; Surgery Chapter 32 VI A*) Congenital dislocation of the hip occurs in 1 per 1000 live births and is much more common in girls and in neonates who were breech presentations. Congenital dislocation of the hip may be bilateral (10%) or unilateral (90%). Most cases can be diagnosed within the first 2 weeks of life, that is, once relaxin has disappeared from the neonate's circulation; however, it may not be diagnosed until the child is about 1 year old. X-rays confirm a suspected diagnosis, and treatment with a Pavlik harness should begin immediately. The aim of the harness is to place the femoral head in the acetabulum and keep it there for about 3 months. Weight bearing in the infant's hip begins at about 6 months when the infant begins to crawl. For children 6 months to 7 years of age with a unilateral congenital hip dislocation and until about 4 years for a bilateral dislocation, it is possible to reduce and splint the hip, thereby obtaining a fair reduction. If closed reduction fails, then open reduction or reconstruction may be necessary.

346. The answer is E (all). (*See Appendix for references*) Carbon monoxide poisoning is best treated by hyperbaric oxygen as this will result in displacement of carbon monoxide by oxygen in the hemoglobin molecule; this will also partially relieve the tissue hypoxia as oxygen is also dissolved in the plasma. Sudden and rapid decompression, as in deep sea divers, results in sequestration of gas bubbles in vascular beds of tissues and organs, leading to hypoxemia. This is also associated with release of fat particles into the circulation. Thus, decompression illness results in air embolism and fat embolism. Hyperbaric oxygen therapy produces impressive, almost immediate improvement in patients with gas gangrene. (Therapy should also include other measures, such as antibiotics and wound debridement). However, hyperbaric oxygen should be used cautiously and intermittently (not continuously).

347. The answer is B (1, 3). [*Medicine Chapter 9 II B 2 d; Preventive Medicine and Public Health Chapter 10 IV A 1 a (4), 2 a (1), 3 e*] Early treatment may prevent mental retardation in phenylketonuria (PKU) and cretinism (hypothyroidism). Mental retardation is prevented in infants with PKU by screening at birth for the presence of PKU and by protecting affected infants from high levels of circulating phenylalanine during the first 5 years of life, using a phenylalanine-free diet. Cretinism is also a congenital disorder characterized by a lack of thyroid secretion. Early detection (i.e., within the first 3 months of life) and administration of thyroid hormone preparations can correct this condition. Down's syndrome is an autosomal anomaly that is not amenable to treatment; the birth of a Down's syndrome infant can be prevented by prenatal screening with amniocentesis and chorionic villus sampling and the subsequent abortion of affected fetuses. Tay-Sachs disease is an autosomal recessive disease that occurs among Ashkenazi Jews. It invariably leads to death within 2 to 4 years as a result of the absence of hexosaminidase A, which leads to the accumulation of gangliosides in the ganglion cells. While screening is available for the identification of Tay-Sachs carriers, no treatment is available for the disease.

348. The answer is A (1, 2, 3). (*Physiology Chapter 3 VIII F 3; see Appendix for references*) The pickwickian syndrome is characterized by obesity, daytime somnolence, *hypercapnia*, hypoxemia, and nocturnal alveolar hypoventilation (sleep apnea). Patients are often morbidly obese, and the somnolence is often striking with patients dozing midsentence. Improvement is dramatic when the patient loses weight.

349. The answer is E (all). (*Medicine Chapter 3 V D 2 a*) Vitamin K, a fat-soluble chemical compound, is necessary for the synthesis of blood coagulation factors II, VII, IX, and X in the liver. The vitamin K that occurs naturally in food is called vitamin K_1. Vitamin K is also synthesized by microorganisms in the gastrointestinal tract; however, because this vitamin is structurally different from vitamin K_1, it is known as vitamin K_2. Synthetic vitamin K is known as vitamin K_3.

350. The answer is E (all). (*Psychiatry Chapter 9 V A 1, 2*) Children who are victims of abuse by parents or guardians usually show pseudomature behavior and signs of physical neglect (e.g., retarded physical growth, malnutrition, or poor hygiene). Any child who presents with unexplained trauma, especially multiple trauma at different stages of healing, should raise the question of abuse. A child who demonstrates the extremes of behavior (e.g., hostility or passivity) or who presents with a recent history of nightmares, phobias, or enuresis should be evaluated for child abuse; this may reflect stress stemming from an abusive situation at home.

351–352. The answers are: 351-A (1, 2, 3), 352-A (1, 2, 3). (*Microbiology Chapter 21 III E 1; Pediatrics Chapter 8 VII E*) The patient in the photograph that accompanies the question presents with a herpes zoster eruption (shingles). This infection occurs predominantly in adults who have had chickenpox (varicella) as a child and who have circulating antibodies. It is characterized by crops of vesicles confined to a dermatome accompanied by pain. Diagnosis is made by clinical presentation and by the Tzanck test, which reveals multinucleated giant cells with intranuclear inclusions. The most common complications of herpes zoster infection include encephalopathy, Guillian-Barré syndrome, aseptic meningitis, and purpura fulminans. Blackwater fever (malaria) is caused by a *Plasmodium falciparum* infection and is associated with hemolysis and hemoglobinuria. Varicella zoster immune globulin is not helpful in the treatment of varicella zoster virus, but it is useful in its prevention, as for example with immunosuppressed patients who have been exposed to this infection.

353. The answer is A (1, 2, 3). *(Psychiatry Chapter 9 III A 3, 4, D 3)* Individuals over the age of 40 years are at greatest risk for suicide. While men *commit* suicide three times more often than women, women *attempt* suicide three times more often than men. The suicide rate is higher for single individuals, especially those divorced or widowed, than for married individuals. A family history of suicide is important in terms of the possibility of inheriting an affective disorder as well as a patient's identification with the individual who died. Unemployed, divorced, Caucasian *men* over the age of 45 years are at especially high risk, but any of these factors occurring singly or in combination should lead a physician to investigate the risk.

354. The answer is B (1, 3). *(Pediatrics Chapter 15 V A 2)* Two defects are responsible for 95% of all cases of congenital adrenal hyperplasia, that is, deficiencies of 21-hydroxylase or 11-hydroxylase. These deficiencies result in hypocortisolism and increased production of adrenocorticotropic hormone (ACTH), which in turn results in adrenocortical hyperplasia and increased production of adrenal androgens (17-ketosteroids). The result is ambiguous genitalia in girls (pseudohermaphroditism) and macrogenitosomia in boys if present during fetal development. Postnatally, it is associated with virilization in prepubertal girls or young women and precocious puberty in boys. It is inherited as an autosomal recessive trait, and it affects boys and girls equally. Treatment involves giving enough glucocorticoid to suppress ACTH, not adrenalectomy. Because there is normal ovarian development in female infants, the internal genital structures are female (see the figure that accompanies the explanation to question 258).

355. The answer is A (1, 2, 3). [*Medicine Chapter 10 III G 3; Pathology Chapter 17 IV C 2 b (2) (c); see also Appendix for references*] The patient in the photograph that accompanies the question is suffering from chronic rheumatoid arthritis. Typically, patients present with joint pain and swelling and limited motion of the affected joint. Subcutaneous rheumatoid nodules are one of the most characteristic findings. Rheumatoid factor (i.e., latex fixation test) is found in 70% to 80% of patients with rheumatoid arthritis, and antinuclear antibodies are found in 25%. Secondary amyloidosis may also be present. The gammaglobulins (e.g., IgM and IgG) are usually elevated as is the erythrocyte sedimentation rate. Amyloidosis is characterized by deposition of a glycoprotein material in various sites in the body, such as smooth muscle, heart, tongue, skin carpal ligaments, and joints. Amyloidosis may be primary or secondary to multiple myeloma, chronic infections, rheumatoid arthritis, ulcerative colitis, and even chronic heroin addiction.

356. The answer is A (1, 2, 3). *(Medicine Chapter 9 III A 4 c, d; see also Appendix for references)* Hypercalcemia causes hyporeflexia, anorexia, nausea, vomiting, constipation, psychosis, and short QT intervals. Sudden death can occur due to asystole or cardiac arrhythmia if serum calcium rises above 12 mg/dl. Hyperreflexia and tetany are caused by hypocalcemia.

357. The answer is A (1, 2, 3). *(Pharmacology, 2nd ed, Chapter 7 III C 3; Surgery Chapter 14 I D 1)* The postphlebitic syndrome occurs in approximately 10% of patients with deep venous thrombosis as a result of obstruction of the deep venous system. This obstruction results in valve damage and venous hypertension, usually following iliofemoral thrombosis. Physical findings include leg edema, pain, abnormal skin pigmentation, and dermatitis. Although fibrinolytic therapy is very expensive, it can decrease the potential for developing postphlebitic syndrome if administered early and appropriately in selected patients.

358. The answer is C (2, 4). *(Obstetrics and Gynecology Chapter 17 V A 1)* A threatened abortion in a patient in early pregnancy is associated with vaginal bleeding or spotting and uterine cramping without cervical dilatation or membrane rupture. While about 20% of patients have some bleeding in pregnancy, only about half of these patients actually have a spontaneous abortion. Inevitable abortion, which is associated with irreversible placental deterioration and a low gonadotropin level, presents with cramps, heavy vaginal bleeding, a dilating cervical canal, and ruptured membranes with or without the products of conception in the cervical canal.

359. The answer is A (1, 2, 3). *(Anatomy Chapter 19 III A 1, 2 b; see also Appendix for references)* A lesion of cauda equina, so-called because it resembles a horse's tail, involves the sacral roots that descend from the lower end of the spinal cord and occupy the vertebral canal below the cord. It may present with root pain, sensory loss, and lower motor neuron paralysis in the distribution of the sacral roots that supply the back of the legs, resulting in sciatica pain and wasting of the hamstring and calf muscles. Knee jerks are increased due to weakness of the opposing hamstrings, and ankle and plantar responses are absent because of sensory loss. There is sensory loss in the buttocks (i.e., saddle area) and urinary retention.

360. The answer is B (1, 3). [*Medicine Chapter 3 I A 3 b, c; Chapter 5 I B 2 c; Pathology Chapter 17 II A 3 a (3) (a) (iii); Psychiatry Chapter 8 IV A, C 2*] In sideroblastic anemia, the red cells are microcytic and hypochromic, but the serum iron is elevated. Iron deposits in the bone marrow, liver, and spleen are excessive. Some of these patients respond to pyridoxine. In thalassemia major, fetal hemoglobin may be increased to 90%. There is a microcytic, hypochromic anemia with target cells. The serum iron is elevated. In pica, non-nutritive substances are eaten for at least 1 month; the disorder is associated with iron deficiency with low serum iron. In Plummer-Vinson syndrome, there is an iron deficiency state that produces koilonychia, dysphagia, glossitis, and other symptoms of anemia, such as fatigue.

361. The answer is E (all). [*Medicine Chapter 3 I C 2 b; Chapter 10 II A 2 a (2)*] Hyperuricemia (serum uric acid >7 mg/dl) may result either from the overproduction or underexcretion of uric acid. Uric acid overproduction may result from increased nucleic acid turnover, as for example, in multiple myeloma, glucose 6-phosphate dehydrogenase deficiency, psoriasis, cancer chemotherapy, and alcohol abuse. Undersecretion of uric acid may be due to the nephrotoxicity of lead poisoning, chronic renal disease, hyper- or hypoparathyroidism, drug effects, organic acid accumulation, and volume depletion states.

362. The answer is A (1, 2, 3). (*Psychiatry Chapter 4 II D 1 c*) Marijuana intoxication produces increased appetite, conjunctival injection, distorted judgment of time and place, euphoria, anxiety, and increased suggestibility, and no change in pupils; it rarely produces hallucinations. Treatment of intoxication involves minimizing the psychological effects, usually by reassuring the patient of eventual recovery. Oral diazepam can be a useful adjunct.

363. The answer is A (1, 2, 3). (*Obstetrics and Gynecology Chapter 17 V A 4; see also Appendix for references*) In missed abortion, the fetus dies in utero, but instead of being expelled, it is retained for 2 months or more. The chorionic gonadotropin levels are low or negative, indicating intrauterine fetal death. In addition, vaginal smears will show a high proportion of cornified cells or sometimes parabasal cells as seen in a postpartal smear. There is a tendency to develop hypofibrinogenemia and disseminated intravascular coagulopathy. The patient often remains amenorrheic throughout this period and thus is usually unaware of the fetal death. Additional symptoms reported by some patients include lassitude, depression, and a peculiar taste in the mouth.

364. The answer is B (1, 3). (*See Appendix for references*) Tuberculoid leprosy can be diagnosed by a positive lepromin skin test. Characteristically, macular lesions with scant bacilli are present, but they are few in number, and they are not symmetric. The patient often presents with the sudden onset of severe nerve involvement; often nerves close to the lesion are palpably enlarged. Muscle atrophy, especially in the hands, results from the neural involvement. Eye involvement (e.g., keratitis), nasal ulcers, epistaxis, anemia, and lymphadenopathy may also occur.

365. The answer is E (all). (*Psychiatry Chapter 3 III J 1, 2, 3 a, b*) The brain uses glucose as the major substrate for metabolic processes, and oxygen is another essential "fuel." Optimal pH, electrolyte concentrations, hydration, and osmolarity are also essential. Any disturbance in these factors can result in impaired cerebral function and present as organic brain syndrome. Uremia and hepatic failure are associated with an acid–base disturbance; hypoglycemia and diabetic ketoacidosis are associated with abnormal glucose metabolism, resulting in organic brain syndrome.

366. The answer is B (1, 3). (*See Appendix for references*) The condition depicted in the picture that accompanies the question is a preauricular sinus with cyst formation due to occlusion of the opening. The cyst often becomes infected, and it may rupture. If the cyst is incised, a cutaneous preauricular ulcer that refuses to heal may follow because the infection is maintained in the sinus. The discharging sinus may be mistaken for tuberculosis. Complete excision of the sinus is curative. The preauricular sinus results from imperfect fusion of the six tubercles that form the pinna. The six tubercles are situated around the posterior end of the first brachial cleft.

367. The answer is A (1, 2, 3). (*Pharmacology, 2nd ed, Chapter 7 III A; Chapter 10 II C; Preventive*

Medicine and Public Health Chapter 5 III C; see also Appendix for references) Well-known risk factors for cerebral thrombosis (stroke) include hypertension, diabetes, hyperlipidemia, and coronary artery disease. Additional risk factors include smoking (especially with hyperlipidemia), thrombocytosis, which is associated with platelet dysfunction that may predispose the patient to thrombosis, and polycythemia, which results in increased viscosity that may also predispose to thrombosis. The incidence of cerebral thrombosis is increased with oral contraceptive use, but age, smoking, and hypertension are important associated risk factors. Heparin, an anticoagulant, is used in the treatment of venous (not arterial) thrombosis; it is not a risk factor for cerebral thrombosis.

368. The answer is B (1, 3). (*Medicine Chapter 1 VII B*) Superficial venous thrombophlebitis, unlike deep venous thrombosis, does not develop embolic complications. Presentation is most often a painful, tender cord in the lower extremities. Management of superficial venous thrombophlebitis includes elevation of the legs, elastic stockings or bandages, heat, and administration of salicylates. Strict bed rest and anticoagulation therapy are not necessary in the management of superficial thrombophlebitis.

369. The answer is E (all). [*Medicine Chapter 5 IX B 2 c (1); Chapter 10 VI B 1; VII B; IX; Pathology Chapter 18 VI A 3 c (3)*] Primary biliary cirrhosis, a disease of unknown etiology, is usually diagnosed between 40–60 years of age. Ninety percent of affected individuals are women. Sjögren's syndrome is an autoimmune disorder that is characterized by dry mouth, dry eyes, and salivary gland enlargement. It is more common in women, especially postmenopausal women, than men. Systemic lupus erythematosus is an autoimmune disorder affecting many organs in the body. It affects young women of childbearing age eight to ten times more often than men. Systemic sclerosis is a connective tissue disorder characterized by small vessel obliterative disease and fibrosis of the skin and multiple other organs. This condition also affects women three to four times more often than men.

370. The answer is E (all). [*Medicine Chapter 1 II A 2 d; Chapter 2 IX C 1; Chapter 5 I B 2 a (1); Pathology Chapter 5 II C 3; see also Appendix for references*] Cigarette smoking is associated with a high incidence of peptic ulcer disease and also cancer of the urinary bladder. Smoking is an etiologic factor in 80% to 85% of cases of bronchogenic cancer and increases the risk of esophageal cancer 2 to 4 times. Thromboangiitis obliterans, a recurrent inflammatory disorder of the arteries associated with thrombosis of medium-sized arteries, occurs almost exclusively in cigarette smokers, especially men between the ages of 25 and 50 years.

371. The answer is A (1, 2, 3). (*Surgery Chapter 9 II D 2*) Oral cholecystography is the most accurate method of demonstrating biliary calculi. (A plain x-ray of the abdomen may show only 15% of gallstones that are radiopaque.) Because this procedure requires ingestion of iopanoic acid tablets, which contain iodine, it is contraindicated if a patient is allergic to iodine. The success of this procedure is also dependent on normal absorption of the contrast material from the gastrointestinal tract, uptake and excretion of the contrast medium from the hepatocytes, uptake and concentration of the contrast medium by the gallbladder, and patency of the hepatic and cystic ducts. Goiter is not a contraindication.

372. The answer is A (1, 2, 3). (*Pediatrics Chapter 5 V C 2 a*) Jaundice, which occurs in 50% of all newborn infants, may be either physiologic or pathologic. Causes of physiologic jaundice—that is, the increased serum concentration of unconjugated bilirubin during the first few days of life—include the delayed activity of glucuronyl transferase, decreased bilirubin clearance from the plasma, and increased bilirubin load on hepatocytes. Pathologic jaundice is hyperbilirubinemia that is secondary to a disease state, such as hemolytic diseases, extravascular blood loss and accumulation (e.g., due to cephalhematoma), increased enterohepatic circulation, breast-feeding associated with poor intake, disorders of bilirubin metabolism, metabolic disorders (e.g., hypothyroidism) bacterial sepsis, prolonged administration of intravenous protein solutions, the TORCH diseases (i.e., toxoplasmosis, other, rubella, cytomegalovirus, and herpes simplex), and neonatal hepatitis. Phenobarbital, which is used in the treatment of hyperbilirubinemia, does not cause neonatal jaundice.

373. The answer is E (all). (*Immunology Chapter 9 V C*) Sensitized T cells (i.e., antigen-reactive cells) react with specific antigens to cause a delayed hypersensitivity reaction. This reaction manifests as an inflammation at the site of the antigen exposure, which normally peaks 24–48 hr after exposure. Delayed hypersensitivity reactions play a very important role in cell-mediated immunity and thus provide resistance to chronic bacterial infections (e.g., tuberculosis), viral infections (e.g., herpes and fungal infections), and tumors, although cytotoxic antibodies may also play a role here, that is, with respect to tumor.

374. The answer is C (2, 4). [*Surgery Chapter 14 I C 3 c (4), d, e*] Deep vein thrombosis is thrombosis in the venous system of the extremities, usually the lower extremities. Venography is the most accurate diagnostic test for deep vein thrombosis. A continuous heparin infusion should begin immediately even if the diagnostic tests have not been completed. Heparin activates antithrombin III, inhibits platelet aggregation, and decreases thrombin availability. Elevation of the extremity reduces edema by aiding venous return, and elastic stockings increase the flow to the deep veins after the patient begins to walk.

375. The answer is E (all). [*Pharmacology, 2nd ed, Chapter 5 I A 8 e (3), (4), (6), 9 f; II H 5 b; Psychiatry Chapter 3 IV F 2 o (1)*] Cardioversion, the conversion of a cardiac arrhythmia to a normal sinus rhythm, is accomplished by applying countershocks to the heart through electrodes placed on the chest wall. This procedure should not be used in sinus tachycardia or arrhythmias (other than ventricular fibrillation) caused by digitalis toxicity. The principal consequence of digitalis overdosage is the initiation and maintenance of tachyarrhythmias. There are also cardiac *effects* of digitalis therapy where the normally upright T wave becomes diminished in amplitude, isoelectric, or inverted in one or more leads. The ST segment may also show *depression* when the QRS complex is *upward*; occasionally, the ST segment is *elevated* by digitalis when the QRS deflection is *downward*. The changes in the ST segment and the T wave may occur alone or may coincide. Propranolol is effective in the treatment of extrasystoles, the most frequent cardiac response to digitalis overdosage, and tachycardia of both ventricular and supraventricular origin; however, it causes a decrease in nodal conduction velocity, which limits its usefulness in the presence of atrioventricular block. Noncardiac symptoms of digitalis intoxication include changes in the gastrointestinal, central nervous, and visual systems. Visual complaints include hazy vision, difficulty in reading, and alterations in the color of objects (chromatopsia) where objects appear green or yellow (xanthopsia). Neural changes include mental confusion, hallucinations, restlessness, insomnia, drowsiness, and, occasionally, overt psychoses.

376. The answer is A (1, 2, 3). [*Medicine Chapter 9 IV A 7 e (1) (b); Pharmacology, 2nd ed, Chapter 3 VII B 2 d (1); Chapter 5 IV F 2 e (2)*] Dopamine is an intermediate in the synthesis of norepinephrine and increases systolic blood pressure with little effect on diastolic blood pressure. Monoamine oxidase (MAO) inhibitors are antidepressants, which form stable complexes with the enzyme MAO, irreversibly inactivating it and thereby preventing oxidative deamination of biogenic amines in the brain, intestines, heart, and blood. However, hypotension, especially postural, can result from the ability of MAO inhibitors to affect ganglionic transmission and reduce the release of norepinephrine in certain organ systems, probably due to uptake and release of "false transmitters," such as tyramine. Prazosin is a selective postsynaptic α_1-adrenergic receptor blocker, causing vasodilatation of both arteries and veins. A significant undesirable effect of prazosin is postural hypotension and syncope, especially if > 1 mg is given. Diabetic autonomic neuropathy may become clinically manifest via postural hypotension, sexual impotence, gastroparesis, and urinary retention.

377. The answer is E (all). (*See Appendix for references*) Hypothermia with a rectal temperature below 35°C may present with drowsiness, delirium, coma, and apnea. Pneumonia, ventricular fibrillation, metabolic acidosis, hypoglycemia or hyperglycemia and renal failure may occur. Electrocardiogram may produce pathognomonic J waves of Osborn. Death usually results from cardiac arrest or ventricular fibrillation. Systemic hypothermia may result from prolonged exposure to extreme cold. Acute alcoholism may be a predisposing factor. Also, patients with cardiovascular or cerebrovascular disease, myxedema, hypopituitarism, and mental retardation are more vulnerable to hypothermia. Administration of large quantities of stored, refrigerated blood (without prewarming) can cause systemic hypothermia.

378. The answer is B (1, 3). (*Psychiatry Chapter III A 2 a, c*) Dementia usually presents with memory difficulties, especially recent (anterograde) memory, which is affected early in this disorder. Remote (retrograde) memory tends to be affected later. Demented patients also present with impaired judgment, emotional lability, and depression. Dementia is also associated with a loss of intellectual abilities of sufficient severity to interfere with occupational and social functioning. It is seen primarily in elderly individuals and affects both the personality and cognitive functioning of the patient. Prolonged heavy ethanol abuse can cause dementia. Clouding of consciousness is a feature of delirium, and although this is not a classic feature of dementia, demented patients are more susceptible to delirium. Visual hallucinations are more characteristic of delirium, but as delirium advances, hallucinations involving any sensory modality may be experienced.

379. The answer is A (1, 2, 3). [*Biochemistry, 2nd ed, Chapter 29 VIII F; Chapter 31 II E 4 a, b; Im-*

munology Chapter 6 II B 2 b (1); Pediatrics Chapter 14 IV C; Pharmacology, 2nd ed, Chapter 11 II B 3, 4, 6; III B] Alkylating agents are antineoplastic compounds that bind covalently to RNA, DNA, and essential proteins of proliferating and nonproliferating cells. Therefore, alkylating agents are phase-nonspecific. Basically, the cytotoxicity of these antitumor agents is related to their effect on guanine, leading to blockage of DNA replication and translation, gene miscoding, and DNA breakage. Mechlorethamine, the prototype of the nitrogen mustards, together with cyclophosphamide and chlorambucil, are alkylating agents. Methotrexate is an antimetabolite that is a folic acid antagonist, which brings about cell death by the inhibition of DNA synthesis through a blockage of thymidylate purine synthesis.

380. The answer is A (1, 2, 3). *[Medicine Chapter 10 IV B 1 d (3) (c) (i)–(iv)]* Ankylosing spondylitis is an inflammatory arthritis that is characterized by inflammation of the axial skeleton, causing backache and limited spinal mobility. Ninety-five percent of white individuals with ankylosing spondylitis have the major histocompatibility antigen (HLA-B27), and forty-five percent of blacks with this disease have this antigen. Low back pain is the most common presenting symptom; it can present as mild morning stiffness or severe and debilitating pain. Ankylosing spondylitis may be complicated by cardiac, pulmonary, and ocular abnormalities. Episodic uveitis occurs in 25% of patients with ankylosing spondylitis. Aortic valve insufficiency often results from inflammation at the root of the aorta, and upper lobe pulmonary fibrosis in severe ankylosing spondylitis can become extensive. Although chronic prostatitis may occur with ankylosing spondylitis, urethritis is not a clinical feature of the disease.

381. The answer is C (2, 4). *[Medicine Chapter 3 V D 2 b (4), d (2)]* Disseminated intravascular coagulopathy is a very common acquired coagulopathy. It is initiated by stimuli in the systemic circulation that activate the coagulation mechanism and cause the abnormal formation of excessive thrombin. The excessive thrombin then activates extensive coagulation in the microcirculation, resulting in the decrease of many coagulation moieties and in secondary activation of the fibrinolytic system. A deficiency of various clotting factors develops, and both the prothrombin time and the partial thromboplastin time are prolonged. Platelet count drops, resulting in thrombocytopenia. Fibrinogen deficiency arises from thrombin-mediated clotting as well as plasmin-mediated fibrinolysis, resulting in the presence of high titers of fibrin degradation products. Specific inhibitors of coagulation are antibodies with specificity for single coagulation proteins. The most common is factor VIII antibody, which arises in approximately 10% of hemophiliacs who have received factor therapy. Diagnosis is made by demonstrating a specific factor deficiency that is not corrected by administration of normal plasma.

382. The answer is E (all). *(Psychiatry Chapter 2 V A 2 a)* Circadian rhythms refer to bodily functions that adhere to 24-hr cycles. The major circadian rhythms that have been identified include REM and non-REM variations in sleep, sleep and wakefulness periods, liver enzymes, cell reproduction and sensitivity, menstrual cycles in women, adrenal steroid secretion, blood pressure, and diurnal variations in mood. Malfunction of these internal rhythms might explain features of an affective illness—for example, difficulty falling asleep, excessive sleep, early morning awakening, and variations in rest–activity cycles.

383. The answer is E (all). *(Medicine Chapter 5 II C 1 b; Surgery Chapter 33 IX A 7; see also Appendix for references)* Congenital pyloric stenosis usually presents in infancy, occurring in 2–4 of 1000 births, and is usually seen in the first born male. It presents clinically with nonbile-stained vomiting that progresses gradually to projectile vomiting. Surgical treatment consists of pyloromyotomy (Fredet-Ramstedt's operation), which involves the incision of the serosa over the pylorus and the division of the hypertrophic muscle of the antrum but not the duodenum. The loss of hydrochloric acid, potassium, and fluid by vomiting can lead to a hypochloremic, hypokalemic alkalosis with dehydration. Preoperative corrective measures include volume repletion, potassium supplementation, and correction of the alkalosis with sodium bicarbonate.

384. The answer is A (1, 2, 3). *(Medicine Chapter 4 X A, C)* Multiple myeloma is an uncommon neoplasm of the plasma cells derived from B lymphocytes. The cardinal feature is the presence of an abnormal "M" protein in the blood or urine. The "M" protein consists of any one or a combination of heavy chains, immunoglobulins G (IgG) and A (IgA), and light chains (i.e., kappa and lambda). Complications of multiple myeloma include infiltration of the bone marrow by large numbers of abnormal plasma cells, pathologic fractures due to osteolytic lesions, which may present radiologically as punched out lesions, hypercalcemia, and amyloid deposits in various organs.

385. The answer is B (1, 3). *(See Appendix for references)* Hemifacial spasm is a benign condition that affects the left side more often than right and women more commonly than men. However, this facial spasm can sometimes progress to cause great physical and psychological stress. Speech and vision on the affected side may become impaired. Anticonvulsant drugs, such as phenytoin and carbamazepine, usually are not helpful.

386. The answer is A (1, 2, 3). [*Surgery Chapter 31 VII C 1 b (3); see also Appendix for references*] The Brown-Séquard syndrome (i.e., hemisection of the spinal cord) is characterized by disease on one side of the spinal cord caused by a tumor compression on the cord or spinal injury. It consists of contralateral sensory (i.e., pain and temperature sensation) loss, ipsilateral proprioceptive loss below the lesion, and ipsilateral motor loss. The ipsilateral motor loss is due to a lesion of the pyramidal (corticospinal) tract. The loss of vibration sense is due to a lesion of the posterior column. The loss of pain and temperature sensation on the opposite side is due to involvement of the spinothalamic tract, which decussates lower down and ascends up this tract. There is no loss of tactile sensation because touch has a double path, one on the same side and one on the opposite side. See the cross section of the spinal cord showing the major sensory pathways below.

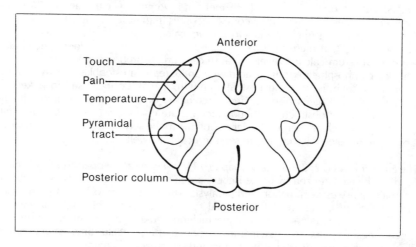

387. The answer is A (1, 2, 3). (*Medicine Chapter 10 II A 1, 2*) Gout, which is characterized by hyperuricemia (uric acid elevation) and urate deposition in tissues, may be caused by thiazide diuretics, cancer chemotherapy, and psoriasis. Diuretics, especially thiazides, cause volume depletion and consequent increased urate resorption with possible decreased uric acid secretion by the tubules. Secondary hyperuricemia is associated with increased nucleic acid turnover, which is, in turn, associated with cancer chemotherapy and psoriasis. Overhydration, which results in dilution of uric acid, will not cause gout. All gouty syndromes are characterized by either episodic or constant elevation of serum urate above 7 mg/dl and urate deposition in articular or extra-articular tissue.

388. The answer is E (all). (*Psychiatry Chapter 9 V A 1, 2*) At least 500,000 children are significantly injured each year as a result of child abuse, and child abuse is underreported in the United States. Characteristics of parents reported for child abuse typically include the following: The parents often overreact to the child's condition, are distrustful, and are uncooperative. There may also be signs of negligence regarding the child's physical hygiene and dress—for example, the child may be inappropriately dressed for the weather.

389. The answer is E (all). [*Medicine Chapter 9 IV A 7 b (1) (a), (b)*] Diabetic retinopathy is related to the duration and severity of diabetes. It is manifested by dark red "dots," hard exudates, dark red "blots," and proliferating new blood vessels. Red "dots," which may not be visible with an ophthalmoscope, are due to small microaneurysms; red "blots," on the other hand, may be due to small hemorrhages or large microaneurysms. Hard exudates are due to lipid accumulation. Proliferative retinopathy is characterized by proliferating new blood vessels and is associated with intraocular hemorrhage and progressive loss of vision.

390. The answer is A (1, 2, 3). (*See Appendix for references*) Neonatal goiter will result if increased levels of thyroid-stimulating hormone are produced because of a defect in the production of T_3 and T_4. This defect can result from an inborn error of metabolism and maternal ingestion of antithyroid drugs or iodine-containing medications (e.g., cough medicines) during pregnancy. Maternal alcoholism is not goitrogenic but can result in the fetal alcohol syndrome, which may be associated with mental retardation.

391. The answer is A (1, 2, 3). (*Medicine Chapter 2 XIV B; Pathology Chapter 11 III C 4*) Goodpasture's syndrome, a disease that affects primarily men in their twenties or thirties, is characterized by progressive renal and lung disease; the etiology is unknown. Lung disease is manifested by intra-alveolar hemorrhage, and the renal lesion is a proliferative glomerulonephritis. Presenting complaints include cough, hemoptysis, and hypochromic iron deficiency anemia. The prognosis is poor, and the patient may eventually need bilateral nephrectomy and renal transplantation.

392. The answer is D (4). (*Medicine Chapter 9 VIII B 3 a; see also Appendix for references*) Senile osteoporosis is characterized by a loss of both cortical and trabecular bone. Vertebral and hip fractures are common. Senile osteoporosis affects both men and women over the age of 75 years. The whole skeleton is equally affected. The bony cortex becomes thinner (as demonstrated on bone scan). The etiology of osteoporosis is unclear, but a low serum calcium is not a characteristic feature; however, it has been postulated that there may be increased bone resorption in elderly individuals in order to maintain normal serum calcium levels because calcium absorption is decreased.

Serum alkaline phosphatase is associated with an increase in osteoblastic activity in normal physiologic conditions, such as fetal and postnatal growth; it may be increased in rickets, osteomalacia, hyperparathyroidism, Paget's disease, and sarcoidosis, or it may be elevated with hepatocellular disease or cholangiolar obstruction. Pseudofractures are characteristic bands of decalcification (seen radiographically), which are perpendicular or oblique to the surface of the bone. These are considered pathognomonic of osteomalacia but are seen in rickets as well.

393. The answer is A (1, 2, 3). (*Surgery Chapter 13 V A–D; see also Appendix for references*) Peripheral vascular disease characterized by acute ischemia due to sudden arterial occlusion or injury may present with pain, pulselessness, pallor, and paralysis. The pallor, cyanosis, and pulselessness result because of the lack of perfusion of tissue distal to the occlusion. This ischemia eventually leads to ischemic necrosis (i.e., gangrene). Risk factors include smoking, hypertension, abnormal lipoproteins, and diabetes mellitus. Shock is not a feature of sudden arterial occlusion of peripheral arterial vessels; shock is seen with coronary arterial occlusion and pancreatic infarction.

394. The answer is A (1, 2, 3). (*Medicine Chapter 6 VII C*) Hypertension is blood pressure exceeding 140/95 mm Hg in men over 45 years of age, 160/95 mm Hg in women over 45 years of age, and 130/90 mm Hg in any adult between 20 and 45 years of age. Rapidly progressive and severe hypertension may be complicated by damage to the brain (e.g., subarachnoid hemorrhage or encephalopathy), heart (e.g., congestive heart failure), retina (e.g., hemorrhage or papilledema), or kidney (e.g., hematuria or azotemia).

395. The answer is E (all). (*Pathology Chapter 18 IV C 1; Surgery Chapter 25 VIII B 1, 2*) Squamous cell carcinoma is the most common epithelial tumor of the larynx. It is found almost exclusively in men who smoke (90%), but as more women smoke, more women have squamous cell carcinoma of the larynx. The combination of heavy smoking and heavy alcohol consumption appears to increase the risk. The most common presenting symptom is hoarseness. Squamous cell carcinoma affects approximately 9000 patients per year in the United States.

396. The answer is A (1, 2, 3). [*Surgery Chapter 9 II E 3 d, F 2 b (1), J 2 a*] Cholelithiasis (gallstones) results from the precipitation of biliary solutes. Acute inflammation of the gallbladder (cholecystitis) is associated with cholelithiasis insofar as obstruction of the cystic duct causes inflammation. Cholelithiasis is more common in women and diabetic individuals, who are at increased risk for complications. It is frequently asymptomatic, although most patients eventually develop symptoms or complications. Approximately 90% of patients with cancer of the gallbladder have a history of cholelithiasis. This condition is frequently seen in the "fair, fat, fertile female."

397. The answer is E (all). (*Psychiatry Chapter 1 II B*) Eugene Bleuler introduced the concept of the four A's in describing the fundamental symptoms of schizophrenia. These are disturbances in: (1) **a**ssociation, where there is incoherence or loosening of associations; (2) **a**ffect, where there is blunted or inappropriate external expression of feelings; (3) **a**mbivalence, where there is erraticism, unpredictability, and conflicting thoughts; and (4) **a**utism, where there is a preoccupation with self. Bleuler believed that hallucinations and delusions were secondary to these four fundamental symptoms.

398. The answer is B (1, 3). [*Medicine Chapter 10 IV B 1 e (4) (b), 2 d*] Reiter's syndrome, a seronegative reactive arthritis, is, like ankylosing spondylitis, associated with the histocompatibility antigen, HLA-B27. Specific infections, such as urethritis (nonspecific) or dysentery, trigger the clinical expression of arthritis. Conjunctivitis and uveitis are also common manifestations. Nephrolithiasis is not associated with Reiter's syndrome, although cardiovascular changes may occur, especially in severe, long-standing disease. Bamboo spine is seen radiographically in patients suffering from ankylosing spondylitis.

399. The answer is A (1, 2, 3). [*Medicine Chapter 2 XIV A 5 a (1), (3) (b)*] Sarcoidosis is a chronic, noncaseating, granulomatous condition that affects the lung primarily but also other organs and tissues, such as bones and joints (e.g., polyarthritis), eyes (e.g., iridocyclitis), and lymph nodes (e.g., lymphadenopathy). It is associated with periarthritis and an inflammatory polyarthritis similar to rheumatoid arthritis early in the course of the disease. Most patients present with polyarthritis erythema nodosum and bilateral hilar adenopathy. Pulmonary involvement, manifesting as cough, fatigue, and exertional dyspnea, is reported in 90% of cases. Involvement of serosal surfaces is a classic manifestation of tuberculosis that is not observed in sarcoidosis.

400. The answer is D (4). (*Psychiatry Chapter 2 VIII A 4 a–c*) Electroconvulsive therapy (ECT) has been used for several decades to treat major depression. The mechanism of action of ECT is unknown, but it is associated with a very low morbidity and mortality. The success rate is greater than 90%. Patients selected for ECT fall into four groups: (1) severely depressed patients with psychomotor retardation, somatic delusions, and persistent suicidal tendencies; (2) patients with a past history of good response to ECT; (3) patients who have not responded to pharmacotherapy or who cannot take antidepressants; and (4) manic patients who have not responded to other therapies.

401. The answer is A (1, 2, 3). (*See Appendix for references*) Erythrasma is a chronic bacterial infection, although it may resemble tinea versicolor or psoriasis. It is caused by *Corynebacterium minutissimum* and manifests as reddish, brown patches on the toe webs, inner thighs, scrotum, or axilla. It is sensitive to broad-spectrum antibiotics, especially erythromycin. It causes a characteristic coral red fluorescence with Wood's light (rays), which is ultraviolet light used to detect fluorescent materials in the skin and hair in certain disease states, such as tinea capitis.

402. The answer is E (all). (*Medicine Chapter 1 III B 3; VI B 1; Chapter 2 X B; see also Appendix for references*) Idiopathic pulmonary hypertension is due to a structural narrowing of the pulmonary arteries; the etiology is unknown. Secondary pulmonary hypertension may be due to progressive obliteration of pulmonary arterioles by repeated thromboses or emboli, or it may be due to a passive rise in pulmonary artery pressure (e.g., due to mitral valve stenosis or left ventricular failure). In a small number of cases, there may be, in addition, active pulmonary vasoconstriction, resulting in a considerable rise in pulmonary artery pressure. Kyphoscoliosis decreases lung volume and mobility, resulting in atelectasis due to pulmonary compression followed by pulmonary hypertension. Secondary pulmonary hypertension may also result from an increased blood flow through the lungs such as in ventricular septal defect.

403. The answer is A (1, 2, 3). [*Biochemistry, 2nd ed, Chapter 28 I B 4; Medicine Chapter 9 V F 4 a–c; Pathology Chapter 15 VI F 1 a, b; Pharmacology, 2nd ed, Chapter 2 II F 1 a (1); Chapter 5 IV G 2 a (1)*] Anxiety and excitement do not elevate the excretion of catecholamines sufficiently to cause diagnostic errors. On the other hand, acute myocardial infarction, surgical trauma, and shock may cause abnormally high urinary output of the catecholamines and their metabolites. Administration of exogenous catecholamines, such as vasopressors, even for nasal congestion (i.e., ephedrine), highly fluorescent compounds (i.e., tetracyclines and quinine), and certain antihypertensive drugs (i.e., methyldopa) may influence the results of catecholamine determinations without an appreciable effect on vanillylmandelic acid determinations. Methyldopa and ephedrine may falsely elevate urinary catecholamine values. Thiazides, clonidine, and ganglionic blockers do not affect urinary catecholamine concentrations.

404. The answer is A (1, 2, 3). (*Medicine Chapter 8 VI D 1 a–d*) Lyme disease has only recently been described (within the past 10 years or so). It is a systemic infection caused by the spirochete, *Borrelia burgdorferi*, which is transmitted by tick bite. It presents as a skin rash (i.e., erythema chronicum migrans), which is diagnostic of the disease. Aseptic meningitis, carditis, or arthritis may develop months after the first presentation. Lyme arthritis, which is indistinguishable from rheumatoid arthritis, responds to either penicillin or tetracycline. The fluorescent treponemal antibody absorption (FTA-ABS) test is specific for *Treponema pallidum* infection; it is also valuable in determining whether a positive non-treponemal antigen test is false-positive or is indicative of syphilis, whereby it remains positive in spite of successful treatment. False-positive FTA-ABS tests occur rarely in systemic lupus erythematosus and in other disorders associated with abnormal globulin.

405. The answer is A (1, 2, 3). (*Medicine Chapter 5 IX C 3; Pathology Chapter 10 III B 3*) Increased absorption of iron, leading to the deposition of iron in the liver, heart, pancreas, and other organs, is known as hemochromatosis. Excessive iron in the pancreas can cause fibrosis and diabetes, and excessive iron in the liver can cause cirrhosis. This condition is thought to be inherited as an autosomal recessive trait. Men are affected more often than women.

406–411. The answers are: 406-B, 407-C, 408-A, 409-B, 410-D, 411-D. [*Pharmacology, 2nd ed, Chapter 3 IV A 1 a–c, B 1 a, b, C 1, 2; Psychiatry Chapter 3 IV F 2 n (1), (2)*] Levodopa, the immediate precursor of dopamine, is therapeutically useful because it can penetrate the blood–brain barrier and elevate brain dopamine levels in patients with parkinsonism. Levodopa, an amino acid, is converted to dopamine by dopa decarboxylase. It remains one of the primary agents in the treatment of Parkinson's disease.

Carbidopa, a dopa decarboxylase inhibitor, does not cross the blood–brain barrier; therefore, the conversion of levodopa to dopamine is inhibited only in the periphery. The coadministration of these two catecholamines allows low doses of levodopa to be administered. Carbidopa, which inhibits dopa decarboxylase in the periphery (i.e., liver and gastrointestinal tract), allows a larger percentage of the administered levodopa to reach its site of action in the brain (i.e., substantia nigra) and in the kidney, where levodopa functions as a neurotransmitter and a vasodilator, respectively.

Neither carbidopa nor levodopa has urinary antiseptic properties, and neither drug is an antiviral agent. However, amantadine, a synthetic antiviral agent that has been used for the treatment and prophylaxis of A_2 (Asian) influenza virus infections and for the treatment of shingles, has mild antiparkinsonian effects.

412–416. The answers are: 412-A, 413-B, 414-D, 415-A, 416-A. [*Behavioral Science Chapter 4 IV A, B 1; Chapter 9 III B 2; Psychiatry Chapter 1 IV B 3 a (1); Chapter 2 VIII A 3; Chapter 3 III A 1 b; IV J 3; Chapter 4 III B 1 g*] Delirium develops over a short period of time, and symptoms include a clouded state of consciousness, disorientation, and perceptual disturbances, especially acute visual hallucinations.

Schizophrenia is a psychosis marked by auditory hallucinations and delusions. There are usually disturbances of the following: (1) associations (i.e., disorganization of thought and speech); (2) affect (i.e., incongruity between ideas and emotion; emotional blunting); (3) ambivalence (i.e., multiple and contradictory feelings to an extreme degree); and (4) autism (i.e., a preoccupation with self). There is no clouding of consciousness.

Lithium carbonate is not useful for the treatment of delirium or schizophrenia. It is the treatment of choice, however, for bipolar (manic depressive) depression.

Sudden barbiturate withdrawal can cause anxiety and agitation, orthostatic hypotension, weakness, tremor, fever, diaphoresis, delirium, which appears on the fourth to seventh days as the syndrome peaks, seizures, and cardiovascular collapse.

Hypoglycemic encephalopathy as a result of a decline in serum glucose concentration may be accompanied by nausea, tachycardia, sweating, hunger, apprehension, and restlessness. As the encephalopathy progresses, disorientation, agitation, confusion, hallucinations, and delirium may occur.

417–420. The answers are: 417-B, 418-B, 419-C, 420-D. [*Medicine Chapter 8 V H 1 d; Pharmacology, 2nd ed, Chapter 12 III A 5, 6 f, k (2) (a), l (3), B 6 b, c (4); see also Appendix for references*] Spectinomycin is available only by injection and is useful against penicillinase-producing *Neisseria gonorrhoeae*. It, therefore, can be used in patients who are allergic to penicillin. The recommended dose is 2 g intramuscularly immediately for uncomplicated gonorrhea and 2 g intramuscularly three times a day for 3 days for disseminated gonorrhea.

Ampicillin (3.5 g) together with probenecid (1 g) is used to treat uncomplicated gonorrhea as a single-dose treatment. Disseminated gonorrhea can be treated with ampicillin (3.5 g) and probenecid (1 g) immediately, followed by ampicillin (0.5 g) four times a day for 7 days.

While both spectinomycin and ampicillin can be used to treat disseminated gonorrhea, ampicillin is not useful if it is a penicillinase-producing strain, in which case spectinomycin can be used. However, resistant strains of *N. gonorrhoeae* are also developing against spectinomycin; thus, the drugs of choice are antibiotics, such as augmentin (i.e., a combination of amoxicillin and clavulanic acid) and second- and third-generation cephalosporins.

Ophthalmia neonatorum is caused by *N. gonorrhoeae*, herpes virus type 2, the etiologic agent of inclusive conjunctivitis, and certain opportunistic bacteria. Silver nitrate (1%) is effective in preventing ophthalmia neonatorum caused by *N. gonorrhoeae*. Ampicillin and spectinomycin are not available in ophthalmic drops or ointment. Penicillin G solution can be instilled in the conjunctivae and is effective in preventing gonococcal ophthalmia neonatorum.

421–426. The answers are: 421-C, 422-D, 423-C, 424-A, 425-A, 426-B. (*Preventive Medicine and Public Health Chapter 12 IV C 1 a, e; Medicine Chapter 2 XIII B 1, 2; see also Appendix for references*). Silicosis is an occupational disease that results from inhalation exposure to silica, a blasting abrasive used in sandblasting, granite cutting, tunneling, mining (e.g., gold mining), and metal casting. Silicosis is associated with chronic lung infections, especially tuberculosis. Radiologically, nodules, hilar adenopathy, peripheral "eggshell" calcification of the lymph nodes, and signs of tuberculosis, if present, are evident. Affected individuals may remain asymptomatic for many years, eventually developing pulmonary hypertension and cor pulmonale.

Asbestosis is an occupational disease that results from inhalation of asbestos, a material used in insulation, roofing materials, and automotive parts. Workers in asbestos mining and manufacturing are at risk. Symptoms and radiologic findings appear after prolonged exposure, and the disease progresses even after the patient is no longer exposed to the offending agent. There is an increased incidence of both bronchogenic carcinoma and malignant mesothelioma even after trivial exposure. Eventually the patient may develop pulmonary hypertension and cor pulmonale.

Shaver's disease, or bauxite pneumoconiosis, results from exposure to aluminum dust, causing fibrosis, hilar adenopathy, and atelectasis.

427–433. The answers are: 427-C, 428-B, 429-A, 430-C, 431-B, 432-A, 433-B. [*Medicine Chapter 2 I E 2 (1), (2); see also Appendix for references*] The predominant pathology of the "pink puffer" is emphysema. The patient sufficiently overcomes bronchopulmonary resistance by increased respiratory effort to ventilate enough alveoli and maintain an adequate exchange of gases at the alveolar capillary membrane, thus forestalling hypoxemia. Although the patient may be dyspneic, there is no cyanosis, sputum production is relatively scant, and the pulmonary arterial pressure is normal. The chest x-ray may show hyperlucent lung fields with scant bronchovascular markings without cardiomegaly. The total lung capacity may be increased, and the residual volume may be greatly increased. The arterial PCO_2 is low or normal, the PO_2 is moderately reduced, and the hematocrit may be normal. The electrocardiogram rarely shows any changes.

The predominant pathology of the "blue bloater" is chronic bronchitis with or without emphysema and airway obstruction by mucus and bronchiolar spasm, fibrosis, and inflammation, resulting in inadequate alveolar ventilation and gas exchange. The arterial PCO_2 is elevated, the PO_2 is markedly decreased, and the hematocrit is often elevated. There may be evidence of increased residual lung volume. Cyanosis is pronounced, and dyspnea is less pronounced. The chest x-ray may show increased bronchovascular markings and cardiomegaly secondary to pulmonary hypertension and cor pulmonale. The electrocardiogram frequently shows abnormalities, for example, right axis deviation and abnormal P waves.

It must be stressed that the above forms of chronic obstructive pulmonary disease represent two clinical entities that may in practice not occur in their classic manner. More often a dual appearance of emphysema and chronic bronchitis is evident.

434–438. The answers are: 434-E, 435-D, 436-C, 437-B, 438-A. [*Microbiology Chapter 6 III A 9; Chapter 10 I A 5, 6; Chapter 15 I H 1, 3; Chapter 16 V; Chapter 17 II H 1, 2 a (1), c; Chapter 22 IV A; Pathology Chapter 16 II D 2 d (3) (b)*] *Erysipelothrix rhusiopathiae* is a gram-positive bacterium widely distributed in animals and decaying organic matter. It causes erysipeloid, which in humans is acquired by traumatic inoculation of this organism into the skin. This cutaneous condition is characterized by a painful, erythematous swelling that progresses from the site of entry. This disease is an occupational hazard among fishermen, butchers, veterinarians, and others who handle animals. It is treated with penicillin, erythromycin, and tetracyclines.

The only significant human pathogen in the rhabdovirus group is rabies. In an infected animal (predominantly dogs, but wild animals too), the virus is secreted in the saliva and is transmitted to man by a bite. Classically, infected patients exhibit restlessness and hydrophobia about 1 month after the bite. The virus may infect neurons throughout the nervous system.

Bacillus anthracis, a gram-positive bacterium, is the causative agent of anthrax in humans and animals. Anthrax primarily affects grazing animals (i.e., herbivores), and humans are accidental hosts who come in contact with animal products (e.g., wool, hide, hair, bone, and skin). The most common form of the disease in the United States is cutaneous anthrax characterized by malignant pustules. This disease can also involve the lungs and gastrointestinal tract. Tissue invasion occurs through minute cuts in the skin, by inhalation, and occasionally by ingestion.

Psittacosis is caused by an intracellular parasite, *Chlamydia psittaci*, which occurs naturally in a variety of wild and domestic birds. Humans acquire the disease by inhaling discharge or dust from contaminated fecal material. Psittacosis is primarily an occupational disease of poultry workers. In humans, the disease manifests as an acute pulmonary infection characterized by fever, headache, malaise, myalgia, and a nonproductive, hacking cough. It is treatable with tetracycline and erythromycin.

Sporotrichosis, caused by the fungus *Sporotrichum schenckii*, is commonly found on rotting vegetation and in the soil and occurs with skin trauma in association with gardening and farming. The local infection consists of a chronic granulomatous condition, involving the skin and superficial lymph nodes, characterized by the formation of abscesses, nodules, and ulcers. The local cutaneous infection is treated with oral potassium iodide, while the visceral form of the disease responds to amphotericin B.

439–443. The answers are: 439-E, 440-D, 441-B, 442-C, 443-A. (*Obstetrics and Gynecology Chapter 24 II B 1; Chapter 26 II A 2, B 1, 3, C 3, G 5 b*) Herpes simplex virus (HSV-1 and HSV-2) is an acute inflammatory disease of the genitalia. Most cases are caused by HSV-2, but 13% of cases are caused by HSV-1. The primary infection is usually acquired from a sexual contact, and recurrent infections are flare-ups of a latent infection, not a reinfection. There appears to be a relationship between cervical carcinoma and HSV-2.

The *Neisseria gonorrhoeae* organism is one of the major causative agents for pelvic inflammatory disease (PID); it may be responsible for as many as 40% of cases of PID seen today. *N. gonorrhoeae* organisms can be seen on Gram stain as gram-negative intracellular diplococci.

Trichomonas vaginalis, caused by the flagellate protozoa, *Trichomonas*, infects the vagina, urethra, and periurethral glands. Patients present with a greenish, grey, frothy discharge that may be accompanied by "strawberry spots" on the cervix and vagina. Diagnosis is confirmed by identification of the highly motile trichomonads under low-power magnification.

Gardnerella vaginalis causes a nonspecific vaginitis that is not associated with *Trichomonas* or *Candida*. The discharge is watery and causes an offensive fishy odor. Diagnosis is made by excluding *Trichomonas* and *Candida* as the infectious agents and by wet-mount preparations that microscopically disclose the presence of "clue cells," which are stippled epithelial cells coated with coccobacillary forms of *G. vaginalis*.

Candida albicans produces a curdy, itchy vaginal discharge; it is seen more frequently in diabetic individuals and individuals on long-term broad-spectrum antibiotics or on long-term systemic steroids.

444–451. The answers are: 444-D, 445-A, 446-C, 447-E, 448-C, 449-B, 450-D, 451-B. [*Medicine Chapter 9 I B 2 a (3), b, c; Obstetrics and Gynecology Chapter 15 II E; Table 15-2; Pharmacology, 2nd ed, Chapter 11 II A 3 b, B 4 b, c, e; III B 1 a, b, 6 b; IV C 2 a–e, 5 a, 6 b, 7 a, D 2 b, c, 4 b, 5 c, 7 a, F 2, 5 b (1), 7 b; Psychiatry Chapter 3 IV F 2 v; Surgery Chapter 16 IV A 4*] Vincristine is a major cytotoxic drug in the management of the leukemias and lymphomas, particularly for the induction of remission and also against a variety of solid tumors. The vinca alkaloids cause the arrest in metaphase of cells entering mitosis. The main toxicity of vincristine is neuropathy, which usually presents as a sensorimotor peripheral neuritis with paresthesia, loss of deep tendon reflexes, and muscular weakness. Vincristine chemotherapy can also lead to hyponatremia due to the syndrome of inappropriate antidiuretic hormone (SIADH) secretion. Hyponatremia is the hallmark of SIADH. Vincristine may stimulate hypothalamic-neurohypophyseal ADH production.

Bleomycin is a glycopeptide antineoplastic drug used in the treatment of squamous cell carcinoma, lymphomas, and testicular cancer. This cytotoxic drug produces both single- and double-strand scission and fragmentation of DNA probably via the formation of superoxide and hydroxyl free radicals. The histopathologic characteristics of the toxicity include a necrosis of type 1 alveolar lining cells, atypical epithelial proliferation of type 2 cells, hyaline membrane formation, and pulmonary interstitial fibrosis.

Cyclophosphamide, the alkylating agent with the broadest range of antineoplastic activity, is used to treat a wide range of hematologic malignancies, non-Hodgkin's lymphomas, and solid tumors. This nitrogen mustard anticancer drug is inactive until it is converted by hepatic enzymes to metabolites, which have cytotoxic activity. A toxicity that is unique to cyclophosphamide is a sterile hemorrhagic cystitis, which can occur with high-dose intravenous or low-dose oral administration. Prolonged chemotherapy with cyclophosphamide can lead to infertility, amenorrhea, and possible mutagenesis and carcinogenesis. Since the alkylating drugs act by damaging DNA and interfering with cell replication, gametogenesis is often severely affected. Almost all men are rendered permanently sterile early in a treatment course. Women are less severely affected, although the span of reproductive life may be shortened by the onset of a premature menopause (amenorrhea).

Doxorubicin, a cytotoxic antibiotic, is one of the most successful antitumor drugs. The intercalation of this anthracycline between base-pairs results in the inhibition of DNA synthesis and DNA-dependent RNA synthesis, together with the production of single-strand breaks in DNA. The anthracycline ring of doxorubicin can form free radicals, which account for the cardiac toxicity as the major problem associated with its use. The acute cardiotoxic effects include transient arrhythmias and depression of myocardial function. The histopathologic correlates of chronic cardiotoxicity are mitochondrial swelling, myofibrillar degeneration, and focal necrosis of myocytes.

In general, antimetabolites (e.g., methotrexate) used in cancer chemotherapy are drugs that are structurally related to naturally occurring compounds, such as vitamins, amino acids, or nucleotides. They act by incorporation into nuclear material or by irreversible combination with cellular enzymes, preventing normal cellular division. Methotrexate, as the folic acid analogue, inhibits dihydrofolate reductase, which is the enzyme that catalyzes the formation of tetrahydrofolate from dihydrofolate. Since tetrahydrofolate is converted to a variety of coenzymes necessary for the synthesis of thymidylate and purines, methotrexate exerts its cytotoxic effect through the inhibition of DNA synthesis. Among the adverse reactions of this folate antagonist are gastrointestinal toxicity in the form of ulcerative mucositis and diarrhea. Methotrexate is a potent teratogen and an abortifacient, but it has a lesser long-term mutagenic and carcinogenic potential than do the alkylating agents (e.g., cyclophosphamide).

452–456. The answers are: 452-E, 453-C, 454-D, 455-C, 456-D. (*Medicine Chapter 1 VI B 1–4, C 1–3, D 3, 5; Pediatrics Chapter 10 IV C 4, D, F*) Coarctation of the aorta involves the narrowing of the aorta just below the origin of the subclavian artery. It may be associated with congenital berry aneurysms of the circle of Willis (15%). Radiologically, one may see rib notching due to the erosion of the ribs by large and tortuous intercostal arteries.

Tetralogy of Fallot accounts for 10% of all congenital cardiac lesions, making it the commonest cyanotic congenital heart disease. Manifestations of this disease consist of pulmonary stenosis, ventricular septal defect, right ventricular hypertrophy, and an overriding aorta that results in a right-to-left shunt. On chest x-ray, while the heart size is normal, there is an uplifted apex and a concavity in the pulmonary segment, which give the heart a boot shape.

The ductus arteriosus, which may remain patent, usually closes at birth or soon afterward, resulting in a shunt from the aorta to the pulmonary artery (left-to-right shunt). Clinical examination may show a "collapsing pulse" with a low diastolic blood pressure. A "machinery murmur" (i.e., a continuous murmur in both systole and diastole often with a short silent interval late in diastole; the murmur is loudest in late systole, obscuring S_2, and fades in diastole) in the second left intercostal space is characteristic. Reversal of blood flow (i.e., the shunt) with the development of pulmonary hypertension can result in dyspnea and cyanosis (i.e., the Eisenmenger reaction).

Ventricular septal defect results in a left-to-right shunt, resulting in increased pulmonary blood flow. Because the right ventricle receives blood from the right atrium *and* the left ventricle, pulmonary hypertension also ensues. Ventricular septal defect may occur alone or with other defects (e.g., tetralogy of Fallot). If spontaneous closure does not occur, surgery may be necessary to prevent pulmonary hypertension. A harsh, holosystolic murmur, heard along the left sternal border, is characteristic.

457–461. The answers are: 457-E, 458-C, 459-B, 460-B, 461-A. [*Medicine Chapter 3 V B 3 a; Chapter 8 VI D 1; Chapter 10 II A 4 b (5) (a); III H 3 a (5) (a), (b); VI H 3*] Scurvy, which is characterized by impaired collagen synthesis, is caused by a vitamin C deficiency. Ascorbic acid (1 g daily) is used to treat scurvy, which may also be associated with subperiosteal hemorrhages, prolonged bleeding time, hemarthrosis, perifollicular bleeding, and interdental gum hyperplasia.

Lyme arthritis, which has only been described within the last 15 years, is caused by the spirochete, *Borrelia burgdorferi*. It is transmitted by a tick bite and presents as a skin rash. It responds to both penicillin and tetracycline.

Hydroxychloroquine is an antimalarial drug that can be used in the treatment of rheumatoid arthritis. While significant side effects are uncommon, nausea, epigastric pain, diarrhea, and retinopathy can occur. Regular ophthalmic examinations are necessary during treatment to detect retinopathy, which is rare but potentially very serious if it does occur.

Rheumatoid arthritis can also be treated with gold injections; however, the injectable form, while effective, can be toxic. Gold is toxic to bone marrow and can cause thrombocytopenia, leukopenia, and aplastic anemia. Gold is also nephrotoxic and can cause membranous glomerulonephritis, resulting in profuse proteinuria. Other side effects include pruritic rashes, oral ulcers, and exfoliative dermatitis. A patient on gold injections must be carefully monitored by clinical examination, especially of the urine and blood.

Acute gouty arthritis can be treated with colchicine. Marked clinical improvement with colchicine is relatively specific for gout, and thus this drug can be used when the diagnosis of gout is suspected on clinical grounds. Colchicine (0.6 mg) is administered hourly by mouth until clinical improvement or toxicity (i.e., nausea, vomiting, and diarrhea) occurs. A maximum dose of 6 mg is recommended. Colchicine may also be administered intravenously.

Osteoarthritis is an age-related deterioration of articular cartilage and underlying bone. It is also called degenerative bone disease. It is most commonly seen in middle-aged, postmenopausal women. While there is no known cause, articular damage can result from wear and tear, age, obesity, inflammation, neuropathy and deposition diseases. Genetics may also play a role. Treatment involves weight reduction, joint conservation, analgesia, and exercise.

462–466. The answers are: 462-D, 463-C, 464-B, 465-A, 466-E. (*Psychiatry Chapter 7 III; IV C 2, 4 a, 6; Chapter 9 V B*) Gender identity with the opposite sex is called transsexualism. Transsexual individuals persistently believe that they belong to the opposite sex but are trapped in the body of their biologic sex of birth.

Transvestism is seen in males who have an intermittent but regular compulsion to dress in women's clothes, ranging from underwear alone to full feminine regalia and even assuming feminine behavior. The patient is easily frustrated if he cannot cross-dress. Transvestites are generally heterosexual and not transsexual and dress in women's clothes to become sexually aroused.

Voyeurism involves sexual gratification from watching sexual acts or naked bodies, particularly the genitals. The voyeur is usually not interested in physical contact with the observed person, but rather masturbates to orgasm while watching. Voyeurism is usually heterosexual in nature.

Compulsive sexual interest in or activity with prepubertal children by an adult who is at least 10 years older than the child is called pedophilia.

Sexual activity between members of a family is called incest. Father– (or stepfather–) daughter incest is the most common type of incest; mother–son incest is less common. As many as 200,000 cases of incest are reported each year, but it is estimated that 90% of cases go unreported.

467–473. The answers are: 467-C, 468-A, 469-D, 470-A, 471-A, 472-C, 473-B. [*Biochemistry, 2nd ed, Chapter 29 IX B 3 a–c; Medicine Chapter 7 V D 2 a (7); Chapter 10 II A 2 b (3) (d), 4 b (5) (a), (d), c (5) (a), d (4) (b) (iii), e (2) (c), (3), B 6 c; Pathology Chapter 19 II B 2 e; Pharmacology, 2nd ed, Chapter 9 II B 7; XI B 1, 3 a, 4 b; D 1, 3, E 2 a, c, 4 a, b (1)*] Colchicine is considered the drug of choice for acute gouty arthritis because it can prevent or abort acute attacks of gout. Unlike many antigout agents, colchicine has a minimal effect on uric acid synthesis and excretion. An acute attack of gout occurs as a result of an inflammatory reaction to the deposition in joint tissue of urate microcrystals, which are phagocytized by infiltrating neutrophil leukocytes. Following the lysosomal disruption within these granulocytes, there is a release of degradative enzymes, microcrystals (which may be rephagocytized), and chemotactic factors, all of which cause local inflammation and pain. The antimitotic action of colchicine could explain the reduction of polymorphonuclear leukocytic mobilization into the inflamed area. Colchicine also inhibits the release of histamine from mast cells and the secretion of insulin from pancreatic β cells. Diarrhea, nausea, vomiting, and abdominal pain are the major untoward effects of this drug. The incidence of gastrointestinal side effects is reduced with the intravenous preparation; however, local extravasation can cause necrosis, and bone marrow suppression can occur with high doses. Such risks are minimized by careful inspection of the intravenous lines, avoidance of colchicine treatment in neutropenic patients, and the use of low doses in patients with liver or renal diseases.

Allopurinol, in contrast to the uricosuric drugs that increase renal urate excretion, inhibits the biosynthesis of uric acid by blocking xanthine oxidase. In man, uric acid is formed primarily by the xanthine oxidase–catalyzed oxidation of hypoxanthine and xanthine, which are the penultimate and ultimate steps in uric acid formation. With the allopurinol-induced reduction of the plasma uric acid concentration, the dissolution of tophi (urate deposit) is facilitated, and the onset or progression of chronic gouty arthritis is prevented. The most common toxic effects of this antigout drug include skin rashes, gastrointestinal upset, hepatotoxicity, and fever. The cutaneous reaction is predominantly a pruritic, erythematous, or maculopapular eruption. Because it causes a pronounced decrease in plasma and urinary uric acid levels and does not depend on renal mechanisms for its efficacy, allopurinol is of particular benefit in patients who have already developed renal obstructions due to urate stones (nephrolithiasis). Urine alkalinization and maintenance of high urine volumes are also important preventive measures.

Appropriate doses of aspirin (acetylsalicylic acid) increase the urinary excretion of urates; thus, the salicylates were once used in acute and chronic gout. The uricosuric action is markedly dependent on the dose. Low doses of salicylates (below 2 g) will decrease urate excretion and elevate plasma urate concentrations, which favor an acute gout attack. Since low doses of aspirin depress uric acid clearance, the uricosuric effects of probenecid and sulfinpyrazone are antagonized.

Therapeutic doses of probenecid block the active reabsorption of uric acid that occurs in the proximal tubules, thereby increasing the excretory rate of urate. Thus, uricosuric drugs have a seemingly paradoxical effect on plasma and urinary uric acid concentrations in that, at therapeutic doses, they decrease plasma levels and increase urinary levels of uric acid. Chronic administration of probenecid will decrease the incidence of acute gouty attacks together with the complications usually associated with hyperuricemia, such as renal damage and tophi deposition. It is not useful in treating acute attacks of gouty arthritis. For best results, probenecid requires that the patient be hydrated (3 L of water per day) prior to and during drug treatment. Since the rise in urinary uric acid may result in nephrolithiasis, the urine should be alkalinized with sodium bicarbonate to increase the aqueous solubility of uric acid. Additionally, alkalinizing the urine serves to promote uric acid excretion by decreasing its passive reabsorption through ion trapping within the tubule. Probenecid can impair the active secretion of a variety of acid compounds, including penicillin, sulfonylureas, indomethacin, sulfonamides, sulfinpyrazone, and 17-ketosteroids.

474–478. The answers are: 474-C, 475-D, 476-A, 477-E, 478-B. [*Medicine Chapter 2 XIII B 1 b, c (2), 2 a, 4 a, b, C 1 a, 2 a; XIV A; see also Appendix for references*] Silicosis results from the inhalation of free crystalline silica, which produces a diffuse fibrotic reaction of the lungs. Silicosis may be complicated by tuberculosis.

Asbestosis results from the inhalation of asbestos fibers, which produces a diffuse interstitial cellular and fibrotic reaction. Asbestosis is characterized by breathlessness, digital clubbing, and rales. Recognized sequelae of sufficient exposure include bronchogenic carcinoma and pleural and peritoneal mesothelioma.

Sarcoidosis, while a systemic disease, involves the lung in 90% of cases. It is characterized by the presence of noncaseating granulomas of the lung and other organs, and it usually presents as mediastinal or hilar lymphadenopathy. Uveitis is a common presentation that may progress to blindness.

Berylliosis is characterized by an acute chemical pneumonitis following exposure to beryllium (e.g., in electronic, ceramic, or space-vehicle industries). Chronic beryllium lung disease is very similar to sarcoidosis insofar as it is a multisystem disease characterized by noncaseating granulomas; however, the eyes are not involved.

Bagassosis is a hypersensitivity pneumonitis, which results from the inhalation of the fibrous residue of sugar cane in which the thermophilic actinomycetes have colonized. This is similar to farmer's lung in which thermophilic actinomycetes grow in moldy hay and are inhaled when the hay is disturbed.

479–483. The answers are: 479-C, 480-A, 481-B, 482-D, 483-D. [*Medicine Chapter 6 Part I XVI A 2 b (3); Pathology Chapter 12 IV E 1; Chapter 13 III B 6 b; Chapter 15 VI F 2; Chapter 20 III A 4, F 6; Pharmacology, 2nd ed, Chapter 10 II D 3; Chapter 11 III B 4 a, b; VI C 4*] Wilm's tumor, a renal tumor that is usually diagnosed before 8 years of age, has metastasized in one-third of patients by the time the diagnosis is made. Treatment by surgical removal of the tumor (nephroblastoma), followed by radiotherapy and adjuvant chemotherapy with actinomycin D, vinblastine, cisplatin, and doxorubicin, has improved the 5-year survival rates, which are now around 60%.

Prostatic carcinoma is most common in men over 50 years of age and in certain racial groups—that is, there is a high prevalence in blacks but a low prevalence in Orientals. Treatment is most often with chemotherapy—diethylstilbestrol or doxorubicin plus cyclophosphamide—but antiandrogenic therapy and radiotherapy are also useful. Surgery is not possible if the tumor has metastasized.

Carcinomas of the adrenal gland (e.g., neuroblastoma) can appear as inoperable tumors. Mitotane selectively destroys normal and neoplastic adrenocortical cells and thus is used as palliative treatment for inoperable adrenal carcinoma.

Choriocarcinomas of gestational origin (50% are preceded by a molar pregnancy, 22% by a normal pregnancy, and 3% by ectopic pregnancy) are rare neoplasms that are potentially curable (75%–80%). Low-risk tumors can be cured with actinomycin D or methotrexate, and metastatic tumors are treated with the above two drugs plus cyclophosphamide. Methotrexate is also useful in the treatment of mycosis fungoides, a cutaneous lymphoproliferative disorder that is progressive, and psoriasis, a disease manifested by white, scaly plaques usually on the elbows and knees.

484–488. The answers are: 484-E, 485-D, 486-C, 487-B, 488-A. [*Medicine Chapter 9 V F 5 a (1) (a) (iii); Pharmacology, 2nd ed, Chapter 5 IV E 3 a (3), c (1), e (3), F 1 a (1), (2), b (2), e (2), 2 e (1), (2), G 1 e (2); Chapter 6 IV A 1–7; Physiology Chapter 5 VII B 2 e*] Nitroprusside is chemically unusual in that it consists of an iron coordination complex with five cyanide moieties and one nitroso group, which give the complex a net negative charge and cause it to associate with two sodium ions (Na^+). This vasodilator, which reduces blood pressure in all patients regardless of body position (i.e., supine or standing) or cause of hypertension, elicits relaxation of vascular smooth muscle in *both* arteries and veins. Nitroprusside must be administered by continuous intravenous infusion. It is inactivated in the liver to cyanide which, in turn, is converted, in the presence of sulfur, to thiocyanate. Thus, a decline in the availability of sulfur will lead to a cyanide toxicity.

Clonidine is a centrally acting antihypertensive drug that stimulates α-adrenergic receptors (i.e., probably presynaptic α_2-receptors) in the vasomotor centers of the brain, resulting in a decreased sympathetic tone to the peripheral vasculature. Following the abrupt withdrawal of clonidine therapy, there ensues a potentially dangerous "rebound hypertension," which appears to be the result of excessive sympathetic nervous activity. This phenomenon may be due, in part, to the development of a hypersensitivity in either the sympathetic nerves or the cardiovascular effector organs (heart and blood vessels).

Prazosin is now classified as a selective α_1-adrenergic (postsynaptic) blocker that causes vasodilation in both arteries and veins. Following the initial oral dose of prazosin, especially if the dose is larger than 1 mg, postural (orthostatic) hypotension and syncope can occur, probably due to the decreased venous return.

Minoxidil is an orally active arteriolar vasodilator agent used for the treatment of severe hypertension that does not respond adequately to more conventional antihypertensive therapy. It decreases renal vascular resistance while preserving renal blood flow and the glomerular filtration rate. A troublesome side effect, particularly in women, is the growth of body hair. This has been suggested to occur because of an increased blood flow to the hair follicles. This particular side effect is currently being investigated as a treatment for baldness.

Acetazolamide is a carbonic anhydrase inhibitor that interferes with the generation of hydrogen ion (H^+) from carbon dioxide and water, leading to a fall in H^+ secretion and bicarbonate ion (HCO_3^-) reabsorption in the proximal and distal convoluted tubules. Since H^+ secretion is retarded, the reabsorption of Na^+ in exchange for the H^+ is also decreased. The inhibition of renal H^+ formation and secretion produces a HCO_3^- diuresis. These effects lead to the formation of an alkaline urine and a systemic hyperchloremic metabolic acidosis. By inhibiting the proximal reabsorption of Na^+, acetazolamide promotes the excretion of a hypotonic urine because the Na^+, which is not reabsorbed proximally, is delivered to the distal diluting sites of the tubule where Na^+ reabsorption is not impaired.

489–492. The answers are: 489-E, 490-D, 491-B, 492-F. (Microbiology Chapter 24 I A 1, 3 b, B 4; II A 5 c; III D 2) The etiologic agents of malaria are Plasmodium falciparum, P. malariae, P. ovale, and P. vivax. These plasmodia occur in the gastrointestinal tract of mosquitoes and are transmitted to humans during a blood meal. Massive intravascular hemolysis can occur in falciparum malaria, resulting in hemoglobinuria, which is referred to as blackwater fever.

Toxoplasma gondii causes a disease, toxoplasmosis, that is similar in clinical presentation to infectious mononucleosis. Symptoms include lymphadenopathy, pharyngitis, fever, rash, and hepatosplenomegaly. In pregnant women, it can pass through the placental barrier to infect the fetus, and because the fetal immune system is not fully developed, it can cause intrauterine fetal death and stillbirths.

Entamoeba histolytica is an amoebic infection that affects the gastrointestinal system. It is spread by the fecal–oral route. Most individuals are asymptomatic, but symptoms include diarrhea, flatulence, and abdominal cramps. Amoebic dysentery is common in debilitated patients. Hepatic abscesses in the upper outer quadrant of the right lobe occur in about 5% of cases.

Trypanosoma cruzi causes South American trypanosomiasis, also known as Chagas' disease. Chagas' disease is a febrile illness associated with cardiac and gastrointestinal involvement. African trypanosomiasis, also known as sleeping sickness, is caused by T. brucei and is associated with panencephalitis. T. brucei is ingested by the tsetse fly and then is transmitted to humans by the bite of the fly; thus, African trypanosomiasis is confined to areas in central Africa where the tsetse fly is endemic.

493–497. The answers are: 493-C, 494-A, 495-B, 496-D, 497-E. [Pathology Chapter 5 II D 1 a, b (3), 2 d; Chapter 16 II A 3 b (1)–(3); see also Appendix for references] The term mycotic aneurysm is a misnomer, as it refers to a bacterial infection of the arterial wall, not a fungal infection. Mycotic aneurysms are associated with bacterial endocarditis and are caused by a weakening of the arterial walls by infected emboli. Sequelae include the spread of infection into the subarachnoid space (i.e., leptomeningitis) and extension into the parenchyma, resulting in an abscess and cerebral hemorrhage.

Syphilitic aneurysms are most commonly found in the aortic arch. Patients present with respiratory difficulty (compression of the trachea), dysphagia (compression of the esophagus), cough and hoarseness (compression of the laryngeal nerve), bone pain (pressure erosion of the ribs), and aortic valvular disease. Syphilitic aneurysms are not seen very often today because tertiary syphilis is now rare.

The most common aneurysm is the atherosclerotic aneurysm. It usually occurs in the internal carotid, vertebral, or basilar arteries where the arterial wall is weakened by severe atheroma and hypertension and is usually fusiform in which the lumen is more or less expanded.

Berry aneurysms are small saccular aneurysms that resemble berries. They are most often congenital and affect the cerebral arteries around the circle of Willis. They become manifest as a subarachnoid hemorrhage.

A false aneurysm is often traumatic in origin; it is essentially an extravascular hematoma that communicates with the lumen of the blood vessel. A true aneurysm is due to dilatation of an artery and may be saccular, fusiform, or dissecting.

498–500. The answers are: 498-E, 499-D, 500-C. [*Behavioral Science Chapter 8 II E 2 b (1)–(3); Psychiatry Chapter 1 IV A 2, 3*] Hallucinations are the perception of an imaginary or interoceptive event as an exteroceptive reality. The type and nature of the misperception may suggest the type of underlying pathology; for example, auditory hallucinations, usually in the form of voices, are characteristic of schizophrenia, while tactile hallucinations are characteristic of withdrawal delirium. Exceptions, however, are very common.

Delusions are fixed, false beliefs based on an incorrect interpretation of reality. Delusions include: overvalued ideas, that is, persistent, unreasonable beliefs that may be considered eccentric rather than pathologic; delusions of reference, which attribute personal significance to the behavior of others or to unrelated external events; delusions of influence or control, in which the individual feels controlled by mysterious forces; and persecutory and grandiose delusions, in which the individual feels persecuted because of grandiose attributes or relationships.

Illusions are misinterpretations or misconceptions of actual environmental events. Examples of illusions are déjà vu, in which a new situation is felt to have been experienced before; jamais vu, in which a familiar situation is experienced as new; distorted perceptions of the passage of time; hypersensitivity to light, sound, or smell; and misperception of movement and perspective.

Appendix: References

AMA Department of Drugs: *Drug Evaluations*, 6th ed. Chicago, American Medical Association, 1986

Anderson JE: *Grant's Atlas of Anatomy*, 8th ed. Baltimore, Williams and Wilkins, 1983

Bates B: *A Guide to Physical Examination and History Taking*, 4th ed. Philadelphia, JB Lippincott, 1987

Berkow R, Fletcher AJ: *The Merck Manual of Diagnosis and Therapy*, 15th ed. Rahway, NJ, Merck, Sharp, and Dohme Research Laboratories, 1987

Braunwald E, Isselbacher KJ, Petersdorf RG, et al: *Harrison's Principles of Internal Medicine*, 11th ed. New York, McGraw-Hill, 1987

Bressman JI, Fahn S: Current concepts in Parkinson's disease. *Hosp Med* November:33–56, 1983

Clain A: *Hamilton Bailey's Demonstrations of Physical Signs in Clinical Surgery*, 17th ed. Bristol, John Wright, 1986

Clemente CD: *Gray's Anatomy*, 30th ed. Philadelphia, Lea and Febiger, 1985

Ellis H, Calne RY: *Lecture Notes on General Surgery*, 6th ed. Oxford, Blackwell Scientific, 1983

Fawcett, DW: *A Textbook of Histology*, 11th ed. Philadelphia, WB Saunders, 1986

Fischer DS: Answers to questions on occult neoplasm. *Hosp Med* September:57–59, 1983

Gage AM, Gage AA: Varicose veins: to treat or not to treat. *Hosp Med* September:97–124, 1983

Gilman AG, Goodman LS, Rall TW, et al: *Goodman and Gilman's Pharmacological Basis of Therapeutics*, 7th ed. New York, Macmillan, 1985

Greene LF: Rational management of prostatitis. *Hosp Med* March:13–31, 1984

Hyperbaric oxygen. (Editorial) *Brit Med J* April:1012, 1978

Klein RJ, Freidman-Kien AE, Hatcher VA: Herpes simplex virus infections: an update. *Hosp Med* November:169–193, 1983

Klingenberg C: Right bundle branch block. *Hosp Med* September:34–46, 1983

Konrad HR: Carcinoma of the larynx. *Hosp Med* August:165–179, 1984

Longcope CP: Adrenogenital syndrome. *Hosp Med* April:79–85, 1984

Lucka BK: Zollinger-Ellison syndrome. *Hosp Med* December:143–147, 1983

Maddrey WC: Axioms on chronic hepatitis. *Hosp Med* June:20–26, 1984

Michael RM, Brown GR: *Drug Consultant, 1985–1986: A Pocket Clinical Guide to Drugs and Their Usefulness*. New York, John Wiley, 1985

Moosa AS: Early detection of breast carcinoma. *Med Dig* 12:8–11, 1986

Newman JC, Hurson G, Lane JM: Osteogenic sarcoma. *Hosp Med* December:113– 131, 1983

Orland MJ, Saltman RJ: *Manual of Medical Therapeutics*, 25th ed. Boston, Little, Brown, 1986

Parmley WW: Athlete's heart syndrome. *Hosp Med* March:27–32, 1985

Pritchard JA, MacDonald PC, Gant NF: *Williams Obstetrics*, 17th ed. Norwalk, CN, Appleton-Century-Crofts, 1985

Rains AJH, Capper WM: *Bailey and Love's Short Practice of Surgery*, 15th ed. London, HK Lewis, 1971

Rapoport S: Common peripheral nerve injuries. *Hosp Med* June:33–59, 1984

Riccardi VM: von Recklinghausen's neurofibromatosis. *N Engl J Med* 302(27):1617–1627, 1981

Robinson R, Stott R: *Medical Emergencies: Diagnosis and Management*. Philadelphia, JB Lippincott, 1976

Rovit RL, Murali R: Hemifacial spasm. *Hosp Med* March:65–71, 1984

Schroeder S, Krupp MA, Tierney LM: *Current Medical Diagnosis and Treatment*. Los Altos, CA, Lange, 1987

Sherman DG: Estrogen therapy and risk of recurrent thrombotic stroke. (Letter) *JAMA* 252:1058, 1984

Swash M, Mason S: *Hutchison's Clinical Methods*, 18th ed. Philadelphia, Bailliere Tindall, 1984

Welch JP: Recognizing and treating acute pancreatitis. *Hosp Med* September:91–118, 1985